Diagnosis within psychiatry necessarily involves consideration of a number of different clinical features. In making a diagnosis, individual psychiatrists tend to vary in the weight they attach to associated psychosocial adversities, or to learning difficulties or to accompanying somatic disease. By dealing with these features on axes that are separate from the psychopathological pattern or syndrome, it has proved possible to record clinically useful information in a manner that is both more comprehensive and more comparable than that in the usual disease category approach.

This volume provides the psychiatric sections of ICD-10 in a multiaxial form that is adapted for ease of use of those dealing with mental disorders in childhood and adolescence. Descriptions have been grouped into axes that have been chosen to provide unambiguous information of maximum clinical usefulness in the greatest number of cases. Building on the popular original framework of four axes, the system has been greatly improved by the inclusion of a new axis for psychosocial situations and by the addition of a further sixth axis on adaptive level, which enables clinicians to code an individual's current level of disability.

Multiaxial classification of child and adolescent psychiatric disorders

The ICD-10 classification of mental and behavioural disorders in children and adolescents

WORLD HEALTH ORGANIZATION

Multiaxial classification of child and adolescent psychiatric disorders

The ICD-10 classification of mental and behavioural disorders in children and adolescents

with an introduction by
PROFESSOR SIR MICHAEL RUTTER

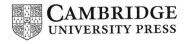

CAMBRIDGE
UNIVERSITY PRESS

PUBLISHED BY THE PRESS SYNDICATE OF THE UNIVERSITY OF CAMBRIDGE
The Pitt Building, Trumpington Street, Cambridge CB2 1RP, United Kingdom

CAMBRIDGE UNIVERSITY PRESS
The Edinburgh Building, Cambridge CB2 2RU, United Kingdom
40 West 20th Street, New York, NY 10011–4211, USA
10 Stamford Road, Oakleigh, Melbourne 3166, Australia

First published 1996

Printed in the United Kingdom at the University Press, Cambridge

Typeset in 10pt Times

A catalogue record for this book is available from the British Library

Library of Congress cataloguing in publication data

World Health Organization.
Multiaxial classification of child and adolescent psychiatric
disorders: the ICD-10 classification of mental and behavioural
disorders in children and adolescents / World Health Organization;
with an introduction by Sir Michael Rutter.
    p. cm.
Includes index.
ISBN 0 521 58133 8 (hardback)
1. Child psychopathology – Classification. 2. Adolescent
psychopathology – Classification. I. Title.
[DNLM: 1. Mental Disorders – classification. 2. Mental Disorders –
in infancy & Childhood. 3. Mental Disorders – in adolescence. WM
15 W927m 1996]
RJ504.W67 1996
618.92'89'0012–dc20
DNLM/DLC
for Library of Congress 96-25102 CIP

ISBN 0 521 58133 8 hardback

Contents

Introduction

by Professor Sir Michael Rutter

Some 25 years ago, a World Health Organization seminar produced findings that argued for a multiaxial approach to the classification of child psychiatric disorder (1). At that time three axes were proposed: clinical psychiatric syndromes, level of intellectual function and associated or etiological factors (physical or environmental). Subsequently, the suggestions included dividing this third axis into its two parts. In 1975, WHO published a report of trials of these four axes, the first three of which were taken from the Eighth Edition of the International Classification of Diseases ICD-8 (2). These trials indicated the increased reliability associated with the use of the axes. Later in 1975 a multiaxial schema was introduced in the United Kingdom adding yet one further axis for specific developmental disorders, which had previously been included with 'biological factors'. This schema was based on the newly introduced ICD-9, with a relatively simple list of associated psychosocial situations. Subsequent studies indicated that the reliability of the psychosocial axis was unacceptably low, and with the prospects that a new edition of the ICD would be appearing in the 1990s, a working group was set up to redraft the psychosocial axis, following the same principles used for the psychiatric disorders in ICD-10. This means that this axis includes a much more detailed specification of the criteria to be used for coding each of the separately identified psychosocial stressors.

This book, then, provides a classification of child and adolescent psychiatric disorders that uses the tenth revision of the International Classification of Diseases (ICD-10), but which places it in a multiaxial framework. The first four axes use precisely the same diagnostic categories as in ICD-10, and the same numerical coding, but the categories have been placed in a somewhat different order so that they fit in with the multi-axial format, and so that those most applicable to children and adolescents appear first. The fifth axis (associated abnormal psychosocial situations) comprises a set of features that are included in ICD-10 as various 'Z' codes, but are set out in much more detail in this book. The development of this axis has been described elsewhere (3). The sixth axis (global assessment of psychosocial disability) is the only one that is not included as such in ICD-10. It has been added here, however, because the assessment of disability has been recognized by WHO as an essential feature in psychiatry (4). The axis is based on the Global Assessment of Disabilities Scale included in the ICD-10 field trials which, in turn, was derived from the fifth axis in DSM-III-R (5). The scale has been slightly modified to make it more appropriate for use with children and adolescents. Its inclusion here should be regarded as a first step towards the development of a systematic scheme for assessing social disability in children and adolescents with psychiatric disorder.

It should be noted that there is a different WHO multiaxial classification for adult psychiatric disorders, comprising just three axes (10).

Principles of a multiaxial framework

Psychiatric diagnosis necessarily involves several different elements. Thus, it may be desirable to note the type of mental disorder, whether or not there is mental retardation, and the presence or absence of associated organic brain disease. In most cases, there is no single diagnostic term that will include all these and it is necessary to use multiple codings. Of course, the ICD makes provision for this but there are no rules as to how many categories to use or the order in which they should be placed. It has been found that, in practice, psychiatrists vary greatly in their use of multiple categories (1, 2). This has the result that when a condition is not coded it may mean that the condition was not present, that it was present but not thought important, or that it was not coded in spite of being thought important. Moreover, there is no way of determining from the coding which was the case.

The multiaxial scheme was designed to remedy these deficiencies. In fact, it is no more than a logical development of the ICD multi-category scheme in which modifications have been introduced specifically to meet the difficulties noted above. To ensure adequate coverage of data, and to ensure comparability, three rules are required: (i) a uniform number of diagnostic elements must be coded (each element having a separate axis); (ii) these codings must always refer to the same elements in diagnosis; and (iii) they must always occur in the same order.

An infinite variety of elements of diagnosis could be included in such a multiaxial scheme, but for it to be workable in practice, there must be a quite restricted number of axes. These need to be chosen on the basis of providing unambiguous information of maximum clinical usefulness in the greatest number of cases. With regard to child and adolescent psychiatry, the axes that were selected refer to the clinical psychiatric syndrome (anorexia nervosa, childhood autism, etc.), to the presence or absence of a specific disorder of psychological development (expressive language disorder, specific reading disorder, etc.), to the intellectual level (normal, mildly retarded, etc.), to medical conditions (cerebral palsy, asthma, etc.), to associated abnormal psychosocial situations (physical child abuse, institutional upbringing, etc.) and to a global assessment of psychosocial functioning (superior/good functioning, moderate impairment, etc.). All items in the first five axes are already in ICD, so that the multiaxial scheme simply regroups the categories under broad headings called `axes'. The sixth axis is an adaptation of an axis in DSM-III-R, and follows the same principles.

The basis of a multiaxial approach is that each of the main elements of diagnosis is systematically recorded on a separate axis, at least one coding being made on each axis for every case. For each axis a no-abnormality coding is provided. For the first four axes these should be coded as 'XX', for Axis Five this is coded as '00' and for Axis Six as '0'. This ensures that there will always be some coding on each of the six axes for every patient and that comparable data on the six elements of diagnosis are coded in the same way and in the same order for all cases, so that systematic data retrieval is a straightforward matter.

The scheme is essentially descriptive and non-theoretical so that it may be used in a comparable fashion by clinicians of differing theoretical persuasion. The aim is to record the presence or absence of different conditions or situations irrespective of whether the clinician considers them to be causal in relation to the psychiatric problem. This procedure is somewhat different from that usually followed in making a diagnostic formulation, but is necessary in view of the continuing theoretical disputes about the importance or otherwise of biological, psychosocial and cognitive factors in etiology.

It should also be emphasized that the codings refer only to a person's current situation and problems and not to the person himself or herself. They carry no implications about permanence or irreversibility, and hence are quite inappropriate for the labelling of individuals (as distinct from the current disorder or situation of that individual). Moreover, the codings for diagnosis on their own can never be the basis for administrative decisions or for institutional placement (which require data on the availability of appropriate treatment, and other features).

Use of the Guide – General

No classification can be used satisfactorily unless some indication is given of the meaning of its constituent terms; that is the purpose of a glossary. However, different degrees of detail and specification are needed for different purposes. The ICD-10 chapter on mental and behavioural disorders comes in three main forms. There is a short version included in the full ICD-10, listing all categories of disease (6). The chapter on mental and behavioural disorders provides relatively brief accounts of the basic concept of each disorder, together with the main diagnostic features. The ICD-10 chapter on mental and behavioural disorders has also been published in two other forms. First, there is a clinical version that provides a more detailed prose description of the concept and diagnostic features relevant to each coding in a set of clinical descriptions and diagnostic guidelines (7). Second, there is a set of diagnostic criteria for research that provides a more structured operationalization of these concepts and features into a set of rules that can be employed in the same way by research workers in different settings (8). This guide has taken the text from the clinical descriptions and diagnostic guidelines for those conditions that are most relevant to children and adolescents. For conditions that are less common in young people, either just a listing of categories is provided, or the text from the short version included in the full ICD-10 is used (6). For research practice, readers must consult the WHO publication of diagnostic criteria for research for this chapter of ICD-10 (8). The criteria provided in this guide for categories in Axis Five, however, are very detailed, and are comparable to 'criteria for research'. They are not available separately.

Axis One:　Clinical Psychiatric Syndromes

The first axis comprises Chapter V 'Mental and Behavioural Disorders' of ICD-10 except that the codes for specific disorders of psychological development have been removed to constitute a second axis; and that the codes for mental retardation have been removed to constitute a separate third axis. Pervasive developmental disorders (F84) are grouped in ICD-10 with specific disorders of psychological development but have been kept in axis one for clinical psychiatric syndromes because that is the usual usage in child and adolescent psychiatry and because it has been strongly preferred by clinicians working in this field. The codings have also been reordered so that the pervasive developmental disorders (F84) and the behavioural and emotional disorders with onset usually occurring in childhood and adolescence (F90–F98) appear first. After that, the order follows that in the ICD-10. The numerical codings and the descriptions of diagnostic categories are unchanged.

It is a principle of ICD-10 that there should not be different classifications for different age groups (although there must be, and is, provision for disorders arising only at particular age periods). As a consequence, the first axis includes codings for disorders that have little relevance for children (e.g. Alzheimer's disease). However, in principle (although only extremely rarely in practice), these diagnoses can apply in childhood and adolescence. Hence, they are included here, and in keeping with the above-mentioned principle of following the order of categories in ICD-10, the dementias and disorders due to psychoactive substance use come early in the book. To facilitate reference, however, the categories that rarely apply to young people are just listed without any description or have been put in smaller type, or are accompanied by briefer descriptions taken from the full ICD-10 (6), rather than the expanded descriptions given in the book devoted to Chapter V (7).

The glossary provides descriptions for all relevant categories but certain general points require emphasis. First, if child psychiatric disorders can be included under one of the headings used with conditions that mainly occur in adult life, that code should be used. Thus, affective disorders are coded the same way irrespective of the age of the subject. Anxiety disorder may, however, be coded under section F40–F48 dealing with a range of anxiety disorders that may arise at any age, or under F93 (emotional disorders with onset specific to childhood). The latter group of disorders are defined in a different way and this code should be used only if the disorder fits the criteria, and not simply because the patient is a child. A full section on disorders of adult personality is included because of their possible applicability in the late adolescence age period and because some clinicians wish to record their early manifestations in childhood (although it is recognized that this is controversial).

Second, although the classification is, in general, based on the principle that assumptions of etiology should be avoided, there are a few exceptions to this principle. Thus, section F00–F09, dealing with 'organic, including symptomatic, mental disorder' groups conditions together on the grounds that they have a demonstrable etiology in cerebral disease, brain injury, or some other insult leading to cerebral dysfunction. Similarly, code F43 is defined in terms of disorder due either to an exceptionally stressful life event producing an acute stress reaction or a significant life change leading to continued unpleasant circumstances that result in an adjustment disorder. Nevertheless, these disorders are defined in terms of the form and pattern of symptomatology and these codings should be used only when disorders meet these criteria. They should not be employed simply because environmental influences are thought to be important in the etiology. Their relevance is catered for in Axis Five.

Finally, it may be noted that there is a special coding (F54) to record the presence of psychological or behavioural influences that are thought to have played a major part in the etiology of physical disorders classified in other chapters (such as asthma or peptic ulcer). If a coding of F54 is made, the relevant physical condition should always be coded separately on the fourth axis.

Axis Two: Specific Disorders of Psychological Development

Codings on this axis are descriptive and not etiological. Specific delays in disorders of psychological development should be coded regardless of their origin (the only exception is that delays solely attributable to poor schooling are excluded). This ruling means that if, for example, a child with childhood autism has a serious impairment in speech or language, this should be coded on this axis. However, to be coded there must be a specific delay in some aspect of development. That is, a child who shows a general delay as part of severe mental retardation should receive a coding of 'XX' on Axis Two (i.e. no specific delay) if the impairment in language is comparable to the degree of impairment in other cognitive functions.

Axis Three: Intellectual Level

This axis provides a description of an individual's current level of general intellectual functioning. If a person is performing at a mentally retarded level, then this should be noted in the coding irrespective of whether the retardation is part of a pervasive developmental disorder, a consequence of sociocultural privation or deprivation, or result of a medical condition such as Down's syndrome. In short, the coding is descriptive and carries no necessary implications concerning either etiology or prognosis. In F70–F79 of Chapter V of ICD-10, the various categories of mental retardation are defined in terms of levels of social functioning. The codes on this axis are parallel to those in F70–F79 but differ in the respect that they are defined strictly in terms of intellectual level (assessed psychometrically or clinically). This is because, for many purposes, it is desirable to have a measure of intellectual level that is independent of social functioning, because the latter may be affected by comorbid conditions on Axis One, and because Axis Six provides a separate global assessment of psychosocial functioning.

Axis Four: **Medical Conditions**

This axis provides for the coding of non-psychiatric medical conditions. The coding refers to current conditions and a past history of illness or injury should not be recorded unless it is associated with some codable current medical condition. However, if a condition is present it should be coded irrespective of whether it is thought to have caused the psychiatric disorder. For the specific codes to be used for particular medical disorders reference should be made to ICD-10 outside Chapter V (6). A brief listing of the broad groups of medical conditions is included here, together with codings for a few specific conditions likely to be of common relevance in psychiatric practice with young people. Acts of self-harm that are associated with a psychiatric disorder should also be recorded in Axis Four by means of an additional X code from ICD-10, Chapter XX. These codes do not allow differentiation between attempted suicide and 'parasuicide', both being included in the general category of self-harm.

Axis Five: **Associated Abnormal Psychosocial Situations**

This axis provides a means of coding abnormal psychosocial situations that *might* be relevant either for causation of psychiatric disorder *or* for therapeutic planning. Because of the latter need, and because of inevitable uncertainties regarding causal inferences, abnormal psychosocial situations should be coded regardless of whether they are thought to have caused the patient's psychiatric disorder.

There is an unavoidable dilemma in decisions on the time frame to which the codings of abnormal psychosocial situations apply. On the one hand, severely adverse experiences in the past may still have current clinical relevance. On the other hand, acute events of a more ordinary kind are likely to be clinically pertinent mainly when they are associated in time with the onset of disorder. Because any building into the codings of a causal inference would open the way to substantial variations among clinicians (and because it would run counter to the generally atheoretical approach of ICD-10), this would constitute an unsatisfactory solution. Accordingly, the codings are expressed here in lifetime terms, but with the recognition that users of the scheme will need to decide for themselves the time frame that best suits their purposes.

Axis Six: **Global Assessment of Psychosocial Disability**

This axis reflects the patient's psychological, social and occupational functioning at the time of the clinical evaluation. It concerns disabilities in functioning that have arisen as a consequence of psychiatric disorder, specific disorders of psychological development or mental retardation. Those that are due to physical (or environmental) limitations should not be coded here.

This axis follows the overall format and subdivisions of the comparable axis in DSM-IV (9). The only modifications are that, as in the scale for the ICD-10 field trials, reference to specific symptoms have been removed (as these are dealt with through Axis One) and slightly more specification is given of the social domains to be taken into account in the coding.

References

1.   Rutter, M., Lebovici L., Eisenberg, L., Sneznevskij, A.V., Sadoun, R., Brooke, E. and Lin, T.Y. (1969). A tri-axial classification of mental disorders in childhood. *Journal of Child Psychology and Psychiatry*, 10, 41–61.

2.   Rutter, M., Shaffer, D. and Shepherd, M. (1975). *An Evaluation of a Proposal for a Multiaxial Classification of Child Psychiatric Disorders*. World Health Organization Monograph. Geneva: World Health Organization.

3.   Van Goor-Lambo, G., Orley, J., Poustka, F. and Rutter, M. (1990). Classification of abnormal psychosocial situations: Preliminary report of a revision of a WHO scheme. *Journal of Child Psychology and Psychiatry*. 31, 229–241.

4.   World Health Organization (1988). *WHO Psychiatric Disability Assessment Schedule (WHO/DAS)*. Geneva: World Health Organization.

5.   American Psychiatric Association (1987). *Diagnostic and Statistical Manual of Mental Disorders – Third Edition – Revised*. Washington DC: American Psychiatric Association.

6. World Health Organization (1991). *International Statistical Classification of Diseases and Health Related Problems.* Tenth Revision. Volume 1. Tabular List. Geneva: World Health Organization.

7. World Health Organization (1992). *The ICD-10 Classification of Mental and Behavioural Disorders. Clinical Descriptions and Diagnostic Guidelines.* Geneva: World Health Organization.

8. World Health Organization (1993). *The ICD-10 Classification of Mental and Behavioural Disorders. Diagnostic Criteria for Research.* Geneva: World Health Organization.

9. American Psychiatric Association (1994). *Diagnostic and Statistical Manual of Mental Disorders.* Fourth Edition. Washington, DC: American Psychiatric Association.

10. Janca, A. (1996). *The Multiaxial Presentation of the ICD-10 for use in Adult Psychiatry.* Published on behalf of the World Health Organization by Cambridge University Press (in press).

Axis One — Clinical Psychiatric Syndromes

List of categories

XX **No psychiatric disorder**

(Code XX when there is no psychiatric disorder of any type falling within Axis One categories. Depending on the computer system used, operators may opt to key in blanks when XX is coded.)

F84 **Pervasive developmental disorders**

F90–F98 **Behavioural and emotional disorders with onset usually occurring in childhood and adolescence**

- F90 Hyperkinetic disorders
- F91 Conduct disorders
- F92 Mixed disorders of conduct and emotions
- F93 Emotional disorders with onset specific to childhood
- F94 Disorders of social functioning with onset specific to childhood and adolescence
- F95 Tic disorders
- F98 Other behavioural and emotional disorders with onset usually occurring in childhood and adolescence

F00–F09 **Organic, including symptomatic, mental disorders**

- F00 Dementia in Alzheimer's disease
- F01 Vascular dementia
- F02 Dementia in other diseases classified elsewhere
- F03 Dementia unspecified
- F04 Organic amnesic syndrome, other than induced by alcohol or other psychoactive substances
- F05 Delirium, other than induced by alcohol and other psychoactive substances
- F06 Other mental disorders due to brain damage or dysfunction or to physical disease
- F07 Personality and behavioural disorders due to brain disease, damage or dysfunction

F09   Unspecified organic or symptomatic mental disorder

F10–F19   **Mental and behavioural disorders due to psychoactive substance use**

F10   Mental and behavioural disorders due to use of alcohol
F11   Mental and behavioural disorders due to use of opioids
F12   Mental and behavioural disorders due to use of cannabinoids
F13   Mental and behavioural disorders due to use of sedatives or hypnotics
F14   Mental and behavioural disorders due to use of cocaine
F15   Mental and behavioural disorders due to use of other stimulants, including caffeine
F16   Mental and behavioural disorders due to use of hallucinogens
F17   Mental and behavioural disorders due to use of tobacco
F18   Mental and behavioural disorders due to use of volatile solvents
F19   Mental and behavioural disorders due to multiple drug use and use of other psychoactive substances

F20–F29   **Schizophrenia, schizotypal and delusional disorders**

F20   Schizophrenia
F21   Schizotypal disorder
F22   Persistent delusional disorders
F23   Acute and transient psychotic disorders
F24   Induced delusional disorder
F25   Schizoaffective disorders
F28   Other nonorganic psychotic disorders
F29   Unspecified nonorganic psychosis

F30–F39   **Mood [affective] disorders**

F30   Manic episode
F31   Bipolar affective disorder
F32   Depressive episode
F33   Recurrent depressive disorder
F34   Persistent mood [affective] disorders
F38   Other mood [affective] disorders
F39   Unspecified mood [affective] disorder

F40–F48   **Neurotic, stress-related and somatoform disorders**

F40   Phobic anxiety disorders

F41	Other anxiety disorders
F42	Obsessive-compulsive disorder
F43	Reaction to severe stress, and adjustment disorders
F44	Dissociative [conversion] disorders
F45	Somatoform disorders
F48	Other neurotic disorders

F50–F59 Behavioural syndromes associated with physiological disturbances and physical factors

F50	Eating disorders
F51	Nonorganic sleep disorders
F52	Sexual dysfunction, not caused by organic disorder or disease
F53	Mental and behavioural disorders associated with the puerperium, not elsewhere classified
F54	Psychological and behavioural factors associated with disorders or diseases classified elsewhere
F55	Abuse of non-dependence-producing substances
F59	Unspecified behavioural syndromes associated with physiological disturbances and physical factors

F60–F69 Disorders of adult personality and behaviour

F60	Specific personality disorders
F61	Mixed and other personality disorders
F62	Enduring personality changes, not attributable to brain damage and disease
F63	Habit and impulse disorders
F64	Gender identity disorders
F65	Disorders of sexual preference
F66	Psychological and behavioural disorders associated with sexual development and orientation
F68	Other disorders of adult personality and behaviour
F69	Unspecified disorder of adult personality and behaviour

F99 Unspecified mental disorder and problems falling short of criteria for any specified mental disorder

List of categories in Axis One with definitions as appropriate

Each group of disorders within Axis One will be dealt with separately, starting with pervasive developmental disorders

F84   **Pervasive developmental disorders**

F84.0   Childhood autism

F84.1   Atypical autism

F84.2   Rett's syndrome

F84.3   Other childhood disintegrative disorder

F84.4   Overactive disorder associated with mental retardation and stereotyped movements

F84.5   Asperger's syndrome

F84.8   Other pervasive developmental disorders

F84.9   Pervasive developmental disorder, unspecified

F84   Pervasive developmental disorders

This group of disorders is characterized by qualitative abnormalities in reciprocal social interactions and in patterns of communication, and by restricted, stereotyped, repetitive repertoire of interests and activities. These qualitative abnormalities are a pervasive feature of the individual's functioning in all situations, although they may vary in degree. In most cases, development is abnormal from infancy and, with only a few exceptions, the conditions become manifest during the first 5 years of life. It is usual, but not invariable, for there to be some degree of general cognitive impairment but the disorders are defined in terms of *behaviour* that is deviant in relation to mental age (whether the individual is retarded or not). There is some disagreement on the subdivision of this overall group of pervasive developmental disorders.

In some cases the disorders are associated with, and presumably due to, some medical condition, of which infantile spasms, congenital rubella, tuberous sclerosis, cerebral lipidosis, and the fragile, X chromosome anomaly are among the most common. However, the disorder should be diagnosed on the basis of the behavioural features, irrespective of the presence or absence of any associated medical conditions; any such associated condition must, nevertheless, be separately coded. If mental retardation is present, it is important that it too should be separately coded, under F70–F79, because it is not a universal feature of the pervasive developmental disorders.

F84.0   Childhood autism

A pervasive developmental disorder defined by the presence of abnormal and/or impaired development that is manifest before the age of 3 years, and by the characteristic type of abnormal functioning in all three areas of social interaction, communication, and restricted, repetitive behaviour. The disorder occurs in boys three to four times more often than in girls.

Diagnostic guidelines

Usually there is no prior period of unequivocally normal development but, if there is, abnormalities become apparent before the age of 3 years. There are always qualitative impairments in reciprocal social interaction. These take the form of an inadequate appreciation of socio-emotional cues, as shown by a lack of responses to other people's emotions and/or a lack of modulation of behaviour according to social context; poor use of social signals and a weak integration of social, emotional, and communicative behaviours; and, especially, a lack of socio-emotional reciprocity. Similarly, qualitative impairments in communications are universal. These take the form of a lack of social usage of whatever language skills are present; impairment in make-believe and social imitative play; poor synchrony and lack of reciprocity in conversational interchange; poor flexibility in language expression and a relative lack of creativity and fantasy in thought processes; lack of emotional response to other people's verbal and nonverbal overtures; impaired use of variations in cadence or emphasis to reflect communicative modulation; and a similar lack of accompanying gesture to provide emphasis or aid meaning in spoken communication.

The condition is also characterized by restricted, repetitive, and stereotyped patterns of behaviour, interests, and activities. These take the form of a tendency to impose rigidity and routine on a wide range of aspects of day-to-day functioning; this usually applies to novel activities as well as to familiar habits and play patterns. In early childhood particularly, there may be specific attachment to unusual, typically non-soft objects. The children may insist on the performance of particular routines in rituals of a nonfunctional character; there may be stereotyped preoccupations with interests such as dates, routes or timetables; often there are motor stereotypies; a specific interest in nonfunctional elements of objects (such as their smell or feel) is common; and there may be a resistance to changes in routine or in details of the personal environment (such as the movement of ornaments or furniture in the family home).

In addition to these specific diagnostic features, it is frequent for children with autism to show a range of other nonspecific problems such as fear/phobias, sleeping and eating disturbances, temper tantrums, and aggression. Self-injury (e.g. by wrist-biting) is fairly common, especially when there is associated severe mental retardation. Most individuals with autism lack spontaneity, initiative, and creativity in the organization of their leisure time and have difficulty applying conceptualizations in decision-making in work (even when the tasks themselves are well within their capacity). The specific manifestation of deficits characteristic of autism change as the children grow older, but the deficits continue into and through adult life with a broadly similar pattern of problems in socialization, communication, and interest patterns. Developmental abnormalities must have been present in the first 3 years for the diagnosis to be made, but the syndrome can be diagnosed in all age groups.

All levels of IQ can occur in association with autism, but there is significant mental retardation in some three-quarters of cases.

Includes:
autistic disorder
infantile autism
infantile psychosis
Kanner's syndrome

Differential diagnosis.
Apart from the other varieties of pervasive developmental disorder it is important to consider: specific developmental disorder of receptive language (F80.2) with secondary socio-emotional problems; reactive attachment disorder (F94.1) or disinhibited attachment disorder (F94.2); mental retardation (F70–F79) with some associated emotional/behavioural disorder; schizophrenia (F20.–) of unusually early onset; and Rett's syndrome (F84.2).

Excludes:
autistic psychopathy (F84.5)

F84.1   ***Atypical autism***
A pervasive developmental disorder that differs from autism in terms *either* of age of onset *or* of failure to fulfil all three sets of diagnostic criteria. Thus, abnormal and/or impaired development becomes manifest for the first time only after age 3 years; and/or there are insufficient demonstrable abnormalities in one or two of the three areas of psychopathology required for the diagnosis of autism (namely, reciprocal social interactions, communication, and restrictive, stereotyped, repetitive behaviour) in spite of characteristic abnormalities in the other area(s). Atypical autism arises most often in profoundly retarded individuals whose very low level of functioning provides little scope for exhibition of the specific deviant behaviours required for the diagnosis of autism; it also occurs in individuals with a severe specific developmental disorder of receptive language. Atypical autism thus constitutes a meaningfully separate condition from autism.

Includes:
atypical childhood psychosis
mental retardation with autistic features

F84.2   ***Rett's syndrome***
A condition of unknown cause, so far reported only in girls, which has been differentiated on the basis of a characteristic onset, course, and pattern of symptomatology. Typically, apparently normal or near-normal early development is followed by partial or complete loss of acquired hand skills and of speech, together with deceleration in head growth, usually with an onset between 7 and 24 months of age. Hand-wringing stereotypies, hyperventilation and loss of purposive hand movements are particularly characteristic. Social and play development are arrested in the first 2 or 3 years, but social interest tends to be maintained. During middle childhood, trunk ataxia and apraxia, associated with scoliosis or kyphoscoliosis tend to develop and sometimes there are choreoathetoid movements. Severe mental handicap invariably results. Fits frequently develop during early or middle childhood.

Diagnostic guidelines
In most cases onset is between 7 and 24 months of age. The most characteristic feature is a loss of purposive hand movements and acquired fine
motor manipulative skills. This is accompanied by loss, partial loss or
lack of development of language; distinctive stereotyped tortuous wring-
ing or 'hand-washing' movements, with the arms flexed in front of the
chest or chin; stereotypic wetting of the hands with saliva; lack of proper
chewing of food; often episodes of hyperventilation; almost always a
failure to gain bowel and bladder control; often excessive drooling and
protrusion of the tongue; and a loss of social engagement. Typically, the
children retain a kind of 'social smile', looking at or 'through' people,
but not interacting socially with them in early childhood (although social
interaction often develops later). The stance and gait tend to become
broad-based, the muscles are hypotonic, trunk movements usually
become poorly coordinated, and scoliosis or kyphoscoliosis usually
develops. Spinal atrophies, with severe motor disability, develop in adolescence or adulthood in about half the cases. Later, rigid spasticity may
become manifest, and is usually more pronounced in the lower than in
the upper limbs. Epileptic fits, usually involving some type of minor
attack, and with an onset generally before the age of 8 years, occur in the
majority of cases. In contrast to autism, both deliberate self-injury and
complex stereotyped preoccupations or routines are rare.

Differential diagnosis.
Initially, Rett's syndrome is differentiated primarily on the basis of the
lack of purposive hand movements, deceleration of head growth, ataxia,
stereotypic 'hand-washing' movements, and lack of proper chewing.
The course of the disorder, in terms of progressive motor deterioration,
confirms the diagnosis.

F84.3   *Other childhood disintegrative disorder*
A pervasive developmental disorder (other than Rett's syndrome) that is
defined by a period of normal development before onset, and by a definite loss, over the course of a few months, of previously acquired skills
in at least several areas of development, together with the onset of characteristic abnormalities of social, communicative, and behavioural functioning. Often there is a prodromic period of vague illness; the child
becomes restive, irritable, anxious, and overactive. This is followed by
impoverishment and then loss of speech and language, accompanied by
behavioural disintegration. In some cases the loss of skills is persistently

progressive (usually when the disorder is associated with a progressive diagnosable neurological condition), but more often the decline over a period of some months is followed by a plateau and then a limited improvement. The prognosis is usually very poor, and most individuals are left with severe mental retardation. There is uncertainty about the extent to which this condition differs from autism. In some cases the disorder can be shown to be due to some associated encephalopathy, but the diagnosis should be made on the behavioural features. Any associated neurological condition should be separately coded.

Diagnostic guidelines
Diagnosis is based on an apparently normal development up to the age of at least 2 years, followed by a definite loss of previously acquired skills; this is accompanied by qualitatively abnormal social functioning. It is usual for there to be a profound regression in, or loss of, language, a regression in the level of play, social skills, and adaptive behaviour, and often a loss of bowel or bladder control, sometimes with a deteriorating motor control. Typically, this is accompanied by a general loss of interest in the environment, by stereotyped, repetitive motor mannerisms, and by an autistic-like impairment of social interaction and communication. In some respects, the syndrome resembles dementia in adult life, but it differs in three key respects: there is usually no evidence of any identifiable organic disease or damage (although organic brain dysfunction of some type is usually inferred); the loss of skills may be followed by a degree of recovery; and the impairment in socialization and communication has deviant qualities typical of autism rather than of intellectual decline. For all these reasons the syndrome is included here rather than under F00–F09.

Includes:
dementia infantilis
disintegrative psychosis
Heller's syndrome
symbiotic psychosis

Excludes:
acquired aphasia with epilepsy (F80.3)
elective mutism (F94.0)
Rett's syndrome (F84.2)
schizophrenia (F20.–)

F84.4   Overactive disorder associated with mental retardation and stereotyped movements

This is an ill-defined disorder of uncertain nosological validity. The category is included here because of the evidence that children with severe mental retardation (IQ below 35) who exhibit major problems in hyperactivity and inattention frequently show stereotyped behaviours; such children tend not to benefit from stimulant drugs (unlike those with an IQ in the normal range) and may exhibit a severe dysphoric reaction (sometimes with psychomotor retardation) when given stimulants; in adolescence the overactivity tends to be replaced by underactivity (a pattern that is *not* usual in hyperkinetic children with normal intelligence). It is also common for the syndrome to be associated with a variety of developmental delays, either specific or global.

The extent to which the behavioural pattern is a function of low IQ or of organic brain damage is not known, neither is it clear whether the disorders in children with mild mental retardation who show the hyperkinetic syndrome would be better classified here or under F90.–; at present they are included in F90.–.

Diagnostic guidelines

Diagnosis depends on the combination of developmentally inappropriate severe overactivity, motor stereotypies, and severe mental retardation; all three must be present for the diagnosis. If the diagnostic criteria for F84.0, F84.1 or F84.2 are met, that condition should be diagnosed instead.

F84.5   Asperger's syndrome

A disorder of uncertain nosological validity, characterized by the same kind of qualitative abnormalities of reciprocal social interaction that typify autism, together with a restricted, stereotyped, repetitive repertoire of interests and activities. The disorder differs from autism primarily in that there is no general delay or retardation in language or in cognitive development. Most individuals are of normal general intelligence but it is common for them to be markedly clumsy; the condition occurs predominantly in boys (in a ratio of about eight boys to one girl). It seems highly likely that at least some cases represent mild varieties of autism, but it is uncertain whether or not that is so for all. There is a strong tendency for the abnormalities to persist into adolescence and adult life and it seems that they represent individual characteristics that are not greatly affected by environmental influences. Psychotic episodes occasionally occur in early adult life.

Diagnostic guidelines

Diagnosis is based on the combination of a lack of any clinically significant general delay in language or cognitive development plus, as with autism, the presence of qualitative deficiencies in reciprocal social interaction and restricted, repetitive, stereotyped patterns of behaviour, interests, and activities. There may or may not be problems in communication similar to those associated with autism, but significant language retardation would rule out the diagnosis.

Includes:
autistic psychopathy
schizoid disorder of childhood

Excludes:
anankastic personality disorder (F60.5)
attachment disorders of childhood (F94.1, F94.2)
obsessive-compulsive disorder (F42.–)
schizotypal disorder (F21)
simple schizophrenia (F20.6)

F84.8   *Other pervasive developmental disorders*

F84.9   *Pervasive developmental disorder, unspecified*
This is a residual diagnostic category that should be used for disorders that fit the general description for pervasive developmental disorders but in which a lack of adequate information, or contradictory findings, means that the criteria for any of the other F84 codes cannot be met.

Behavioural and emotional disorders with onset usually occurring in childhood or adolescence

F90   Hyperkinetic disorders
    F90.0   Disturbance of activity and attention
    F90.1   Hyperkinetic conduct disorder
    F90.8   Other hyperkinetic disorders
    F90.9   Hyperkinetic disorder, unspecified

F91   Conduct disorders
    F91.0   Conduct disorder confined to the family context
    F91.1   Unsocialized conduct disorder
    F91.2   Socialized conduct disorder
    F91.3   Oppositional defiant disorder
    F91.8   Other conduct disorders
    F91.9   Conduct disorder, unspecified

F92   Mixed disorders of conduct and emotions
    F92.0   Depressive conduct disorder
    F92.8   Other mixed disorders of conduct and emotions
    F92.9   Mixed disorder of conduct and emotions, unspecified

F93   Emotional disorders with onset specific to childhood
    F93.0   Separation anxiety disorder of childhood
    F93.1   Phobic anxiety disorder of childhood
    F93.2   Social anxiety disorder of childhood
    F93.3   Sibling rivalry disorder
    F93.8   Other childhood emotional disorders
    F93.9   Childhood emotional disorder, unspecified

F94   Disorders of social functioning with onset specific to childhood and adolescence
    F94.0   Elective mutism
    F94.1   Reactive attachment disorder of childhood
    F94.2   Disinhibited attachment disorder of childhood
    F94.8   Other childhood disorders of social functioning
    F94.9   Childhood disorder of social functioning, unspecified

F95   Tic disorders
    F95.0   Transient tic disorder
    F95.1   Chronic motor or vocal tic disorder
    F95.2   Combined vocal and multiple motor tic disorder [de la Tourette's syndrome]

F95.8   Other tic disorders

F95.9   Tic disorder, unspecified

F98   Other behavioural and emotional disorders with onset usually occurring in childhood and adolescence

F98.0   Nonorganic enuresis

F98.1   Nonorganic encopresis

F98.2   Feeding disorder of infancy and childhood

F98.3   Pica of infancy and childhood

F98.4   Stereotyped movement disorders

F98.5   Stuttering [stammering]

F98.6   Cluttering

F98.8   Other specified behavioural and emotional disorders with onset usually occurring in childhood and adolescence

F98.9   Unspecified behavioural and emotional disorders with onset usually occurring in childhood and adolescence

F90   Hyperkinetic disorders

This group of disorders is characterized by: early onset; a combination of overactive, poorly modulated behaviour with marked inattention and lack of persistent task involvement; and pervasiveness over situations and persistence over time of these behavioural characteristics.

It is widely thought that constitutional abnormalities play a crucial role in the genesis of these disorders, but knowledge on specific etiology is lacking at present. In recent years the use of the diagnostic term 'attention deficit disorder' for these syndromes has been promoted. It has not been used here because it implies a knowledge of psychological processes that is not yet available, and it suggests the inclusion of anxious, preoccupied, or 'dreamy' apathetic children whose problems are probably different. However, it is clear that, from the point of view of behaviour, problems of inattention constitute a central feature of these hyperkinetic syndromes.

Hyperkinetic disorders always arise early in development (usually in the first 5 years of life). Their chief characteristics are lack of persistence in activities that require cognitive involvement, and a tendency to move from one activity to another without completing any one, together with disorganized, ill-regulated, and excessive activity. These problems usually persist through school years and even into adult life, but many affected individuals show a gradual improvement in activity and attention.

Several other abnormalities may be associated with these disorders. Hyperkinetic children are often reckless and impulsive, prone to accidents, and find themselves in disciplinary trouble because of unthinking (rather than deliberately defiant) breaches of rules. Their relationships with adults are often socially disinhibited, with a lack of normal caution and reserve; they are unpopular with other children and may become isolated. Cognitive impairment is common, and specific delays in motor and language development are disproportionately frequent.

Secondary complications include dissocial behaviour and low self-esteem. There is accordingly considerable overlap between hyperkinesis and other patterns of disruptive behaviour such as'unsocialized conduct disorder'. Nevertheless, current evidence favours the separation of a group in which hyperkinesis is the main problem.

Hyperkinetic disorders are several times more frequent in boys than in girls. Associated reading difficulties (and/or other scholastic problems) are common.

Diagnostic guidelines

The cardinal features are impaired attention and overactivity: both are necessary for the diagnosis and should be evident in more than one situation (e.g. home, classroom, clinic).

Impaired attention is manifested by prematurely breaking off from tasks and leaving activities unfinished. The children change frequently from one activity to another, seemingly losing interest in one task because they become diverted to another (although laboratory studies do not generally show an unusual degree of sensory or perceptual distractibility). These deficits in persistence and attention should be diagnosed only if they are excessive for the child's age and IQ.

Overactivity implies excessive restlessness, especially in situations requiring relative calm. It may, depending upon the situation, involve the child running and jumping around, getting up from a seat when he or she was supposed to remain seated, excessive talkativeness and noisiness, or fidgeting and wriggling. The standard for judgement should be that the activity is excessive in the context of what is expected in the situation and by comparison with other children of the same age and IQ. This behavioural feature is most evident in structured, organized situations that require a high degree of behavioural self-control.

The associated features are not sufficient for the diagnosis or even necessary, but help to sustain it. Disinhibition in social relationships, recklessness in situations involving some danger, and impulsive flouting of social rules (as shown by intruding on or interrupting others' activities, prematurely answering questions before they have been completed, or difficulty in waiting turns) are all characteristic of children with this disorder.

Learning disorders and motor clumsiness occur with undue frequency, and should be noted separately (under F80–F89) when present; they should not, however, be part of the actual diagnosis of hyperkinetic disorder.

Symptoms of conduct disorder are neither exclusion nor inclusion criteria for the main diagnosis, but their presence or absence constitutes the basis for the main subdivision of the disorder(see below).

The characteristic behaviour problems should be of early onset (before age 6 years) and long duration. However, before the age of school entry, hyperactivity is difficult to recognize because of the wide normal variation: only extreme levels should lead to a diagnosis in preschool children.

Diagnosis of hyperkinetic disorder can still be made in adult life. The grounds are the same, but attention and activity must be judged with reference to developmentally appropriate norms. When hyperkinesis was present in childhood, but has disappeared and been succeeded by another condition, such as dissocial personality disorder or substance abuse, the current condition rather than the earlier one is coded.

Differential diagnosis

Mixed disorders are common, and pervasive developmental disorders take precedence when they are present. The major problems in diagnosis lie in differentiation from conduct disorder: when its criteria are met, hyperkinetic disorder is diagnosed with priority over conduct disorder. However, milder degrees of overactivity and inattention are common in conduct disorder. When features of both hyperactivity and conduct disorder are present, and the hyperactivity is pervasive and severe, 'hyperkinetic conduct disorder' (F90.1) should be the diagnosis.

A further problem stems from the fact that overactivity and inattention, of a rather different kind from that which is characteristic of a hyperkinetic disorder, may arise as a symptom of anxiety or depressive disorders. Thus, the restlessness that is typically part of an agitated depressive disorder should not lead to a diagnosis of a hyperkinetic disorder. Equally, the restlessness that is often part of severe anxiety should not lead to the diagnosis of a hyperkinetic disorder. If the criteria for one of the anxiety disorders (F40.–, F41.–, F43.–, or F93.–) are met, this should take precedence over hyperkinetic disorder unless there is evidence, apart from the restlessness associated with anxiety, for the additional presence of a hyperkinetic disorder. Similarly, if the criteria for a mood disorder (F30–F39) are met, hyperkinetic disorder should not be diagnosed in addition simply because concentration is impaired and there is psychomotor agitation. The double diagnosis should be made only when symptoms that are not simply part of the mood disturbance clearly indicate the separate presence of a hyperkinetic disorder.

Acute onset of hyperactive behaviour in a child of school age is more probably due to some type of reactive disorder (psychogenic or organic), manic state, schizophrenia, or neurological disease (e.g. rheumatic fever).

Excludes:
anxiety disorders (F41.– or F93.0)
mood [affective] disorders (F30–F39)
pervasive developmental disorders (F84.–)
schizophrenia (F20.–)

F90.0   *Disturbance of activity and attention*
There is continuing uncertainty over the most satisfactory subdivision of hyperkinetic disorders. However, follow-up studies show that the outcome in adolescence and adult life is much influenced by whether or not there is associated aggression, delinquency, or dissocial behaviour. Accordingly, the main subdivision is made according to the presence or absence of these associated features. The code used should be F90.0 when the overall criteria for hyperkinetic disorder (F90.–) are met but those for F91.– (conduct disorders) are not.

Includes:
attention deficit disorder or syndrome with hyperactivity
attention deficit hyperactivity disorder

Excludes:
hyperkinetic disorder associated with conduct disorder (F90.1)

F90.1   *Hyperkinetic conduct disorder*
This coding should be used when both the overall criteria for hyperkinetic disorders (F90.–) *and* the overall criteria for conduct disorders (F91.–) are met.

F90.8   Other hyperkinetic disorders

F90.9   Hyperkinetic disorder, unspecified
This residual category is not recommended and should be used only when there is a lack of differentiation between F90.0 and F90.1 but the overall criteria for F90.– are fulfilled.

Includes:
hyperkinetic reaction or syndrome of childhood or adolescence NOS

F91   Conduct disorders

Conduct disorders are characterized by a repetitive and persistent pattern of dissocial, aggressive, or defiant conduct. Such behaviour, when at its most extreme for the individual, should amount to major violations of age-appropriate social expectations, and is therefore more severe than ordinary childish mischief or adolescent rebelliousness. Isolated disso-cial or criminal acts are not in themselves grounds for the diagnosis, which implies an enduring pattern of behaviour.

Features of conduct disorder can also be symptomatic of other psy-chiatric conditions, in which case the underlying diagnosis should be coded.

Disorders of conduct may in some cases proceed to dissocial person-ality disorder (F60.2). Conduct disorder is frequently associated with adverse psychosocial environments, including unsatisfactory family relationships and failure at school, and is more commonly noted in boys. Its distinction from emotional disorder is well validated; its separation from hyperactivity is less clear and there is often overlap.

Diagnostic guidelines
Judgements concerning the presence of conduct disorder should take into account the child's developmental level. Temper tantrums, for example, are a normal part of a 3-year-old's development and their mere presence would not be grounds for diagnosis. Equally, the violation of other people's civic rights (as by violent crime) is not within the capacity of most 7-year-olds and so is not a necessary diagnostic criterion for that age group.

Examples of the behaviours on which the diagnosis is based include the following: excessive levels of fighting or bullying; cruelty to animals or other people; severe destructiveness to property; fire-setting; stealing;

repeated lying; truancy from school and running away from home; unusually frequent and severe temper tantrums; defiant provocative behaviour; and persistent severe disobedience. Any one of these categories, if marked, is sufficient for the diagnosis, but isolated dissocial acts are not.

Exclusion criteria include uncommon but serious underlying conditions such as schizophrenia, mania, pervasive developmental disorder, hyperkinetic disorder, and depression.

This diagnosis is not recommended unless the duration of the behaviour described above has been 6 months or longer.

Differential diagnosis.
Conduct disorder overlaps with other conditions. The coexistence of emotional disorders of childhood (F93.–) should lead to a diagnosis of mixed disorder of conduct and emotions (F92.–). If a case also meets the criteria for hyperkinetic disorder (F90.–), that condition should be diagnosed instead. However, milder or more situation-specific levels of overactivity and inattentiveness are common in children with conduct disorder, as are low self-esteem and minor emotional upsets; neither excludes the diagnosis.

Excludes:
conduct disorders associated with emotional disorders (F92.–) or hyperkinetic disorders (F90.–)
mood [affective] disorders (F30–F39)
pervasive developmental disorders (F84.–)
schizophrenia (F20.–)

F91.0 Conduct disorder confined to the family context
This category comprises conduct disorders involving dissocial or aggressive behaviour (and not merely oppositional, defiant, disruptive behaviour) in which the abnormal behaviour is entirely, or almost entirely, confined to the home and/or to interactions with members of the nuclear family or immediate household. The disorder requires that the overall criteria for F91 be met; even severely disturbed parent–child relationships are not of themselves sufficient for diagnosis. There may be stealing from the home, often specifically focused on the money or possessions of one or two particular individuals. This may be accompanied by deliberately destructive behaviour, again often focused on specific family members – such as breaking of toys or ornaments, tearing of

clothes, carving on furniture, or destruction of prized possessions. Violence against family members (but not others) and deliberate fire-setting confined to the home are also grounds for the diagnosis.

Diagnostic guidelines

Diagnosis requires that there be no significant conduct disturbance outside the family setting *and* that the child's social relationships outside the family be within the normal range.

In most cases these family-specific conduct disorders will have arisen in the context of some form of marked disturbance in the child's relationship with one or more members of the nuclear family. In some cases, for example, the disorder may have arisen in relation to conflict with a newly arrived step-parent. The nosological validity of this category remains uncertain, but it is possible that these highly situation-specific conduct disorders do not carry the generally poor prognosis associated with pervasive conduct disturbances.

F91.1 Unsocialized conduct disorder

This type of conduct disorder is characterized by the combination of persistent dissocial or aggressive behaviour (meeting the overall criteria for F91 and not merely comprising oppositional, defiant, disruptive behaviour), with a significant pervasive abnormality in the individual's relationships with other children.

Diagnostic guidelines

The lack of effective integration into a peer group constitutes the key distinction from 'socialized' conduct disorders and this has precedence over all other differentiations. Disturbed peer relationships are evidenced chiefly by isolation from and/or rejection by or unpopularity with other children, and by a lack of close friends or of lasting empathic, reciprocal relationships with others in the same age group. Relationships with adults tend to be marked by discord, hostility, and resentment. Good relationships with adults can occur (although usually they lack a close, confiding quality) and, if present, do *not* rule out the diagnosis. Frequently, but not always, there is some associated emotional disturbance (but, if this is of a degree sufficient to meet the criteria of a mixed disorder, the code F92.– should be used).

Offending is characteristically (but not necessarily) solitary. Typical behaviours comprise: bullying, excessive fighting, and (in older children) extortion or violent assault; excessive levels of disobedience, rudeness, uncooperativeness, and resistance to authority; severe temper tantrums and uncontrolled rages; destructiveness to property, fire-setting, and cruelty to animals and other children. Some isolated children, however, become involved in group offending. The nature of the offence is therefore less important in making the diagnosis than the quality of personal relationships.

The disorder is usually pervasive across situations but it may be most evident at school; specificity to situations other than the home is compatible with the diagnosis.

Includes:
conduct disorder, solitary aggressive type
unsocialized aggressive disorder

F91.2   *Socialized conduct disorder*
This category applies to conduct disorders involving persistent dissocial or aggressive behaviour (meeting the overall criteria for F91 and not merely comprising oppositional, defiant, disruptive behaviour) occurring in individuals who are generally well integrated into their peer group.

Diagnostic guidelines
The key differentiating feature is the presence of adequate, lasting friendships with others of roughly the same age. Often, but not always, the peer group will consist of other youngsters involved in delinquent or dissocial activities (in which case the child's socially unacceptable conduct may well be approved by the peer group and regulated by the subculture to which it belongs). However, this is not a necessary requirement for the diagnosis: the child may form part of a non-delinquent peer group with his or her dissocial behaviour taking place outside this context. If the dissocial behaviour involves bullying in particular, there may be disturbed relationships with victims or some other children. Again, this does not invalidate the diagnosis provided that the child has some peer group to which he or she is loyal and which involves lasting friendships.

Relationships with adults in authority tend to be poor but there may be good relationships with others. Emotional disturbances are usually minimal. The conduct disturbance may or may not include the family setting but if it is confined to the home the diagnosis is excluded. Often the disorder is most evident outside the family context and specificity to the school (or other extrafamilial setting) is compatible with the diagnosis.

Includes:
conduct disorder, group type
group delinquency
offences in the context of gang membership
stealing in company with others
truancy from school

Excludes:
gang activity without manifest psychiatric disorder (Z03.2)

F91.3 *Oppositional defiant disorder*

This type of conduct disorder is characteristically seen in children below the age of 9 or 10 years. It is defined by the *presence* of markedly defiant, disobedient, provocative behaviour and by the *absence* of more severe dissocial or aggressive acts that violate the law or the rights of others. The disorder requires that the overall criteria for F91 be met: even severely mischievous or naughty behaviour is not in itself sufficient for diagnosis. Many authorities consider that oppositional defiant patterns of behaviour represent a less severe type of conduct disorder, rather than a qualitatively distinct type. Research evidence is lacking on whether the distinction is qualitative or quantitative. However, findings suggest that, in so far as it is distinctive, this is true mainly or only in younger children. Caution should be employed in using this category, especially in the case of older children. Clinically significant conduct disorders in older children are usually accompanied by dissocial or aggressive behaviours that go beyond defiance, disobedience, or disruptiveness, although, not infrequently, they are preceded by oppositional defiant disorders at an earlier age. The category is included to reflect common diagnostic practice and to facilitate the classification of disorders occurring in young children.

Diagnostic guidelines

The essential feature of this disorder is a pattern of persistently negativistic, hostile, defiant, provocative, and disruptive behaviour, which is clearly outside the normal range of behaviour for a child of the same age in the same sociocultural context, and which does not include the more serious violations of the rights of others as reflected in the aggressive and dissocial behaviour specified for categories F91.0 and F91.2. Children with this disorder tend frequently and actively to defy adult requests or rules and deliberately to annoy other people. Usually they tend to be angry, resentful, and easily annoyed by other people whom they blame for their own mistakes or difficulties. They generally have a low frustration tolerance and readily lose their temper. Typically, their defiance has a provocative quality, so that they initiate confrontations and generally exhibit excessive levels of rudeness, uncooperativeness, and resistance to authority.

Frequently, this behaviour is most evident in interactions with adults or peers whom the child knows well, and signs of the disorder may not be evident during a clinical interview.

The key distinction from other types of conduct disorder is the *absence* of behaviour that violates the law and the basic rights of others, such as theft, cruelty, bullying, assault, and destructiveness. The definite presence of any of the above would exclude the diagnosis. However, oppositional defiant behaviour, as outlined in the paragraph above, is often found in other types of conduct disorder. If another type (F91.0–F91.2) is present, it should be coded in preference to oppositional defiant disorder.

Excludes:
conduct disorders including overtly dissocial or aggressive behaviour
(F91.0–F91.2)

F91.8 Other conduct disorders

F91.9 Conduct disorder, unspecified
This residual category is not recommended and should be used only for disorders that meet the general criteria for F91 but that have not been specified as to subtype or that do not fulfil the criteria for any of the specified subtypes.

Includes:
childhood behavioural disorder NOS
childhood conduct disorder NOS

F92 Mixed disorders of conduct and emotions

This group of disorders is characterized by the combination of persistently aggressive, dissocial, or defiant behaviour with overt and marked symptoms of depression, anxiety, or other emotional upsets.

Diagnostic guidelines
The severity should be sufficient that the criteria for both conduct disorders of childhood (F91.–) and emotional disorders of childhood (F93.–), or for an adult-type neurotic disorder (F40–48) or mood disorder (F30–39) are met.

Insufficient research has been carried out to be confident that this category should indeed be separate from conduct disorders of childhood. It is included here for its potential etiological and therapeutic importance and its contribution to reliability of classification.

F92.0   *Depressive conduct disorder*
This category requires the combination of conduct disorder of childhood (F91.–) with persistent and marked depression of mood, as evidenced by symptoms such as excessive misery, loss of interest and pleasure in usual activities, self-blame, and hopelessness. Disturbances of sleep or appetite may also be present.

Includes:
conduct disorder (F91.–) associated with depressive disorder (F30–F39)

F92.8   *Other mixed disorders of conduct and emotions*
This category requires the combination of conduct disorder of childhood (F91.–) with persistent and marked emotional symptoms such as anxiety, fearfulness, obsessions or compulsions, depersonalization or derealization, phobias, or hypochondriasis. Anger and resentment are features of conduct disorder rather than of emotional disorder; they neither contradict nor support the diagnosis.

Includes:
conduct disorder (F91.–) associated with emotional disorder (F93.–) or neurotic disorder (F40–F48)

F92.9   *Mixed disorder of conduct and emotions, unspecified*

F93   Emotional disorders with onset specific to childhood

In child psychiatry a differentiation has traditionally been made between emotional disorders specific to childhood and adolescence and adult-type neurotic disorders. There have been four main justifications for this differentiation. First, research findings have been consistent in showing that the majority of children with emotional disorders go on to become normal adults: only a minority show neurotic disorders in adult life. Conversely, many adult neurotic disorders appear to have an onset in adult life without significant psychopathological precursors in child-hood. Hence there is considerable discontinuity between emotional dis-orders occurring in these two age periods. Second, many emotional dis-orders in childhood seem to constitute exaggerations of normal developmental trends rather than phenomena that are qualitatively abnormal in themselves. Third, related to the last consideration, there has often been the theoretical assumption that the mental mechanisms involved in emotional disorders of childhood may not be the same as for adult neuroses. Fourth, the emotional disorders of childhood are less clearly demarcated into supposedly specific entities such as phobic dis-orders or obsessional disorders.

The third of these points lacks empirical validation, and epidemiolog-ical data suggest that, if the fourth is correct, it is a matter of degree only (with poorly differentiated emotional disorders quite common in both childhood and adult life). Accordingly, the second feature (i.e. develop-mental appropriateness) is used as the key diagnostic feature in defining the difference between the emotional disorders with an onset specific to childhood (F93.–) and the neurotic disorders (F40–F49). The validity of this distinction is uncertain, but there is some empirical evidence to sug-gest that the developmentally appropriate emotional disorders of child-hood have a better prognosis.

F93.0   *Separation anxiety disorder of childhood*

It is normal for toddlers and preschool children to show a degree of anxi-ety over real or threatened separation from people to whom they are attached. Separation anxiety disorder should be diagnosed only when fear over separation constitutes the focus of the anxiety and when such anxiety arises during the early years. It is differentiated from normal separation anxiety when it is of such severity that is statistically unusual (including an abnormal persistence beyond the usual age period) and when it is associated with significant problems in social functioning. In addition, the diagnosis requires that there should be no generalized dis-turbance of personality development of functioning; if such a distur-bance is present, a code from F40–F48 should be considered. Separation anxiety that arises at a developmentally inappropriate age (such as dur-ing adolescence) should not be coded here unless it constitutes an abnor-mal continuation of developmentally appropriate separation anxiety.

Diagnostic guidelines
The key diagnostic feature is a focused excessive anxiety concerning separation from those individuals to whom the child is attached (usually parents or other family members), that is not merely part of a generalized anxiety about multiple situations. The anxiety may take the form of:

(a) an unrealistic, preoccupying worry about possible harm befalling major attachment figures or a fear that they will leave and not return;

(b) an unrealistic, preoccupying worry that some untoward event, such as the child being lost, kidnapped, admitted to hospital, or killed, will separate him or her from a major attachment figure;

(c) persistent reluctance or refusal to go to school because of fear about separation (rather than for other reasons such as fear about events at school);

(d) persistent reluctance or refusal to go to sleep without being near or next to a major attachment figure;

(e) persistent inappropriate fear of being alone, or otherwise without the major attachment figure, at home during the day;

(f) repeated nightmares about separation;

(g) repeated occurrence of physical symptoms (nausea, stomachache, headache, vomiting, etc.) on occasions that involve separation from a major attachment figure, such as leaving home to go to school;

(h) excessive, recurrent distress (as shown by anxiety, crying, tantrums, misery, apathy, or social withdrawal) in anticipation of, during, or immediately following separation from a major attachment figure.

Many situations that involve separation also involve other potential stressors or sources of anxiety. The diagnosis rests on the demonstration that the common element giving rise to anxiety in the various situations is the circumstance of separation from a major attachment figure. This arises most commonly, perhaps, in relation to school refusal (or 'phobia'). Often, this does represent separation anxiety but sometimes (especially in adolescence) it does not. School refusal arising for the first time in adolescence should not be coded here unless it is primarily a function of separation anxiety, and that anxiety was first evident to an abnormal degree during the preschool years. Unless those criteria are met, the syndrome should be coded in one of the other categories in F93 or under F40–F48.

Excludes:
mood [affective] disorders (F30–F39)
neurotic disorders (F40–F48)

phobic anxiety disorder of childhood (F93.1)
social anxiety disorder of childhood (F93.2)

F93.1   *Phobic anxiety disorder of childhood*

Children, like adults, can develop fear that is focused on a wide range of objects or situations. Some of these fears (or phobias), for example agoraphobia, are not a normal part of psychosocial development. When such fears occur in childhood they should be coded under the appropriate category in F40–F48.However, some fears show a marked developmental phase specificity and arise (in some degree) in a majority of children; this would be true, for example, of fear of animals in the preschool period.

Diagnostic guidelines

This category should be used only for developmental phase-specific fears when they meet the additional criteria that apply to all disorders in F93, namely that:

(a)   the onset is during the developmentally appropriate age period;
(b)   the degree of anxiety is clinically abnormal; and
(c)   the anxiety does not form part of a more generalized disorder.

Excludes:
generalized anxiety disorder (F41.1)

F93.2   *Social anxiety disorder of childhood*

A wariness of strangers is a normal phenomenon in the second half of the first year of life and a degree of social apprehension or anxiety is normal during early childhood when children encounter new, strange, or socially threatening situations. This category should therefore be used only for disorders that arise before the age of 6 years, that are both unusual in degree and accompanied by problems in social functioning, and that are not part of some more generalized emotional disturbance.

Diagnostic guidelines

Children with this disorder show a persistent or recurrent fear and/or avoidance of strangers; such fear may occur mainly with adults, mainly with peers, or with both. The fear is associated with a normal degree of selective attachment to parents or to other familiar persons. The avoidance or fear of social encounters is of a degree that is outside the normal limits for the child's age and is associated with clinically significant problems in social functioning.

One

Includes:
avoidant disorder of childhood or adolescence

F93.3 ***Sibling rivalry disorder***

A high proportion, or even a majority, of young children show some degree of emotional disturbance following the birth of a younger (usually immediately younger) sibling. In most cases the disturbance is mild, but the rivalry or jealousy set up during the period after the birth may be remarkably persistent.

Diagnostic guidelines

The disorder is characterized by the combination of:

(a) evidence of sibling rivalry and/or jealousy;
(b) onset during the months following the birth of the younger (usually immediately younger) sibling;
(c) emotional disturbance that is abnormal in degree and/or persistence and associated with psychosocial problems.

Sibling rivalry/jealousy may be shown by marked competition with siblings for the attention and affection of parents; for this to be regarded as abnormal, it should be associated with an unusual degree of negative feelings. In severe cases this may be accompanied by overt hostility, physical trauma and/or maliciousness towards, and undermining of, the sibling. In lesser cases, it may be shown by a strong reluctance to share, a lack of positive regard, and a paucity of friendly interactions.

The emotional disturbance may take any of several forms, often including some regression with loss of previously acquired skills (such as bowel or bladder control) and a tendency to babyish behaviour. Frequently, too, the child wants to copy the baby in activities that provide for parental attention, such as feeding. There is usually an increase in confrontational or oppositional behaviour with the parents, temper tantrums, and dysphoria exhibited in the form of anxiety, misery, or social withdrawal. Sleep may become disturbed and there is frequently increased pressure for parental attention, such as at bedtime.

Includes:
sibling jealousy

Excludes:
peer rivalries (non-sibling) (F93.8)

F93.8 *Other childhood emotional disorders*

Includes:
identity disorder
overanxious disorder
peer rivalries (non-sibling)

Excludes:
gender identity disorder of childhood (F64.2)

F93.9 *Childhood emotional disorder, unspecified*

Includes:
childhood emotional disorder NOS

F94 Disorders of social functioning with onset specific to childhood and adolescence

This is a somewhat heterogeneous group of disorders, which have in common abnormalities in social functioning that begin during the developmental period, but that (unlike the pervasive developmental disorders) are not primarily characterized by an apparently constitutional social incapacity or deficit that pervades all areas of functioning. Serious environmental distortions or privations are commonly associated and are thought to play a crucial etiological role in many instances. There is no marked sex differential. The existence of this group of disorders of social functioning is well recognized, but there is uncertainty regarding the defining diagnostic criteria, and also disagreement regarding the most appropriate subdivision and classification.

F94.0 *Elective mutism*

The condition is characterized by a marked, emotionally determined selectivity in speaking, such that the child demonstrates his or her language competence in some situations but fails to speak in other (definable) situations. Most frequently, the disorder is first manifest in early childhood; it occurs with approximately the same frequency in the two sexes, and it is usual for the mutism to be associated with marked personality features involving social anxiety, withdrawal, sensitivity, or resistance. Typically, the child speaks at home or with close friends and is mute at school or with strangers, but other patterns (including the converse) can occur.

Diagnostic guidelines

The diagnosis presupposes:

(a) a normal, or near-normal, level of language comprehension;

(b) a level of competence in language expression that is sufficient for social communication;

(c) demonstrable evidence that the individual can and does speak normally or almost normally in some situations.

However, a substantial minority of children with elective mutism have a history of either some speech delay or articulation problems. The diagnosis may be made in the presence of such problems provided that there is adequate language for effective communication and a *gross* disparity in language usage according to the social context, such that the child speaks fluently in some situations but is mute or near-mute in others. There should also be demonstrable failure to speak in some social situations but not in others. The diagnosis requires that the failure to speak is persistent over time and that there is a consistency and predictability with respect to the situations in which speech does and does not occur.

Other socio-emotional disturbances are present in the great majority of cases but they do not constitute part of the necessary features for diagnosis. Such disturbances do not follow a consistent pattern, but abnormal temperamental features (especially social sensitivity, social anxiety, and social withdrawal) are usual and oppositional behaviour is common.

Includes:
selective mutism

Excludes:
pervasive developmental disorders (F84.–)
schizophrenia (F20.–)
specific developmental disorders of speech and language (F80.–)
transient mutism as part of separation anxiety in young children (F93.0)

F94.1   *Reactive attachment disorder of childhood*

This disorder, occurring in infants and young children, is characterized by persistent abnormalities in the child's pattern of social relationships, which are associated with emotional disturbance and reactive to changes in environmental circumstances. Fearfulness and hypervigilance that do not respond to comforting are characteristic, poor social interaction with peers is typical, aggression towards the self and others is very frequent, misery is usual, and growth failure occurs in some cases. The syndrome probably occurs as a direct result of severe parental neglect, abuse, or serious mishandling. The existence of this behavioural pattern is well recognized and accepted, but there is continuing uncertainty regarding the diagnostic criteria to be applied, the boundaries of the syndrome, and whether the syndrome constitutes a valid nosological entity. However, the category is included here because of the public health importance of the syndrome, because there is no doubt of its existence, and because the behavioural pattern clearly does not fit the criteria of other diagnostic categories.

Diagnostic guidelines

The key feature is an abnormal pattern of relationships with care-givers that developed before the age of 5 years, that involves maladaptive features not ordinarily seen in normal children, and that is persistent yet reactive to sufficiently marked changes in patterns of rearing.

Young children with this syndrome show strongly contradictory or ambivalent social responses that may be most evident at times of partings and reunions. Thus, infants may approach with averted look, gaze strongly away while being held, or respond to care-givers with a mixture of approach, avoidance, and resistance to comforting. The emotional disturbance may be evident in apparent misery, a lack of emotional responsiveness, withdrawal reactions such as huddling on the floor, and/or aggressive responses to their own or others' distress. Fearfulness and hypervigilance (sometimes described as 'frozen watchfulness') that are unresponsive to comforting occur in some cases. In most cases, the children show interest in peer interactions but social play is impeded by negative emotional responses. The attachment disorder may also be accompanied by a failure to thrive physically and by impaired physical growth (which should be coded according to the appropriate somatic category (R62) in Axis Four).

Many normal children show insecurity in the pattern of their selective attachment to one or other parent, but this should not be confused with the reactive attachment disorder, which differs in several crucial respects. The disorder is characterized by an abnormal type of insecurity shown in markedly contradictory social responses not ordinarily seen in normal children. The abnormal responses extend across different social situations and are not confined to a dyadic relationship with a particular care-giver; there is a lack of responsiveness to comforting; and there is associated emotional disturbance in the form of apathy, misery, or fearfulness.

Five main features differentiate this condition from pervasive developmental disorders. First, children with a reactive attachment disorder

One

have a normal capacity for social reciprocity and responsiveness, whereas those with a pervasive developmental disorder do not. Second, although the abnormal patterns of social responses in a reactive attachment disorder are initially a general feature of the child's behaviour in a variety of situations, they remit to a major degree if the child is placed in a normal rearing environment that provides continuity in responsive care-giving. This does not occur with pervasive developmental disorders. Third, although children with reactive attachment disorders may show impaired language development (of the type described under F80.1), they do not exhibit the abnormal qualities of communication characteristic of autism. Fourth, unlike autism, reactive attachment disorder is not associated with persistent and severe cognitive deficits that do not respond appreciably to environmental change. Fifth, persistently restricted, repetitive, and stereotyped patterns of behaviour, interests and activities are not a feature of reactive attachment disorders.

Reactive attachment disorders nearly always arise in relation to grossly inadequate child care. This may take the form of psychological abuse or neglect (as evidenced by harsh punishment, persistent failure to respond to the child's overtures, or grossly inept parenting), or of physical abuse or neglect (as evidenced by persistent disregard of the child's basic physical needs, repeated deliberate injury, or inadequate provision of nutrition). Because there is insufficient knowledge of the consistency of association between inadequate child care and the disorder, the presence of environmental privation and distortion is not a diagnostic requirement. However, there should be caution in making the diagnosis in the absence of evidence of abuse or neglect. Conversely, the diagnosis should not be made automatically on the basis of abuse or neglect: not all abused or neglected children manifest the disorder.

Excludes:
Asperger's syndrome (F84.5)
disinhibited attachment disorder of childhood (F94.2)
maltreatment syndromes, resulting in physical problems (T74)
normal variation in pattern of selective attachment
sexual or physical abuse in childhood, resulting in psychosocial problems (Z61.4–Z61.6)

F94.2 *Disinhibited attachment disorder of childhood*
A particular pattern of abnormal social functioning that arises during the first 5 years of life and that, having become established, shows a tenden-

cy to persist despite marked changes in environmental circumstances. At age about 2 years it is usually manifest by clinging and diffuse, non-selectively focused attachment behaviour. By age 4 years, diffuse attachments remain but clinging tends to be replaced by attention-seeking and indiscriminately friendly behaviour. In middle and later childhood, individuals may or may not have developed selective attachments but attention-seeking behaviour often persists, and poorly modulated peer interactions are usual; depending on circumstances, there may also be associated emotional or behavioural disturbance. The syndrome has been most clearly identified in children reared in institutions from infancy but it also occurs in other situations; it is thought to be due in part to a persistent failure of opportunity to develop selective attachments as a consequence of extremely frequent changes in care-givers. The conceptual unity of the syndrome depends on the early onset of diffuse attachments, continuing poor social interactions, and lack of situation-specificity.

Diagnostic guidelines
Diagnosis should be based on evidence that the child showed an unusual degree of diffuseness in selective attachments during the first 5 years *and* that this was associated with generally clinging behaviour in infancy and/or indiscriminately friendly, attention-seeking behaviour in early or middle childhood. Usually there is difficulty in forming close, confiding relationships with peers. There may or may not be associated emotional or behavioural disturbance (depending in part on the child's current circumstances). In most cases there will be a clear history of rearing in the first years that involved marked discontinuities in care-givers or multiple changes in family placements (as with multiple foster family placements).

Includes:
affectionless psychopathy
institutional syndrome

Excludes:
Asperger's syndrome (F84.5)
hospitalism in children (F43.2)
hyperkinetic or attention deficit disorder (F90.–)
reactive attachment disorder of childhood (F94.1)

F94.8 *Other childhood disorders of social functioning*

Includes:
disorders of social functioning with withdrawal and shyness due to social competence deficiencies

F94.9 *Childhood disorder of social functioning, unspecified*

F95 Tic disorders

The predominant manifestation in these syndromes is some form of tic. A tic is an involuntary, rapid, recurrent, non-rhythmic motor movement (usually involving circumscribed muscle groups), or vocal production, that is of sudden onset and serves no apparent purpose. Tics tend to be experienced as irresistible but they can usually be suppressed for varying periods of time. Both motor and vocal tics may be classified as either simple or complex, although the boundaries are not well defined. Common simple motor tics include eye-blinking, neck-jerking, shoulder-shrugging, and facial grimacing. Common simple vocal tics include throat-clearing, barking, sniffing, and hissing. Common complex tics include hitting one's self, jumping, and hopping. Common complex vocal tics include the repetition of particular words, and sometimes the use of socially unacceptable (often obscene) words (coprolalia), and the repetition of one's own sounds or words (palilalia).

There is immense variation in the severity of tics. At the one extreme the phenomenon is near-normal, with perhaps 1 in 5 to 1 in 10 children showing transient tics at some time. At the other extreme, Tourette's syndrome is an uncommon, chronic, incapacitating disorder. There is uncertainty about whether these extremes represent different conditions or are opposite ends of the same continuum; many authorities regard the latter as more likely. Tic disorders are substantially more frequent in boys than in girls and a family history of tics is common.

Diagnostic guidelines
The major features distinguishing tics from other motor disorders are the sudden, rapid, transient, and circumscribed nature of the movements, together with the lack of evidence of underlying neurological disorder; their repetitiveness; (usually) their disappearance during sleep; and the ease with which they may be voluntarily reproduced or suppressed. The lack of rhythmicity differentiates tics from the stereotyped repetitive movements seen in some cases of autism or of mental retardation.

Manneristic motor activities seen in the same disorders tend to comprise more complex and variable movements than those usually seen with tics. Obsessive-compulsive activities sometimes resemble complex tics but differ in that their form tends to be defined by their purpose (such as touching some object or turning a number of times) rather than by the muscle groups involved; however, the differentiation is sometimes difficult.

Tics often occur as an isolated phenomenon but not infrequently they are associated with a wide variety of emotional disturbances, especially, perhaps, obsessional and hypochondriacal phenomena. However, specific developmental delays are also associated with tics.

There is no clear dividing line between tic disorder with some associated emotional disturbance and an emotional disorder with some associated tics. However, the diagnosis should represent the major type of abnormality.

F95.0 Transient tic disorder
Meets the general criteria for a tic disorder, but tics do not persist for longer than 12 months. This is the commonest form of tic and is most frequent about the age of 4 or 5 years; the tics usually take the form of eye-blinking, facial grimacing, or head-jerking. In some cases the tics occur as a single episode but in other cases there are remissions and relapses over a period of months.

F95.1 Chronic motor or vocal tic disorder
Meets the general criteria for a tic disorder, in which there are motor or vocal tics (but not both); tics may be either single or multiple (but usually multiple), and last for more than a year.

F95.2 Combined vocal and multiple motor tic disorder [de la Tourette's syndrome]
A form of tic disorder in which there are, or have been, multiple motor tics and one or more vocal tics, although these need not have occurred concurrently. Onset is almost always in childhood or adolescence. A history of motor tics before development of vocal tics is common; the symptoms frequently worsen during adolescence, and it is common for the disorder to persist into adult life.

The vocal tics are often multiple with explosive repetitive vocalizations, throat-clearing, and grunting, and there may be the use of obscene words or phrases. Sometimes there is associated gestural echopraxia,

One

which also may be of an obscene nature (copropraxia). As with motor tics, the vocal tics may be voluntarily suppressed for short periods, be exacerbated by stress, and disappear during sleep.

F95.8 Other tic disorders

F95.9 Tic disorder, unspecified

A non-recommended residual category for a disorder that fulfils the general criteria for a tic disorder but in which the specific subcategory is not specified or in which the features do not fulfil the criteria for F95.0, F95.1 or F95.2.

F98 Other behavioural and emotional disorders with onset usually occurring in childhood and adolescence

This rubric comprises a heterogeneous group of disorders that share the characteristic of onset in childhood but otherwise differ in many respects. Some of the conditions represent well defined syndromes, but others are no more than symptom complexes which lack nosological validity, but which are included because of their frequency and association with psychosocial problems, and because they cannot be incorporated into other syndromes.

Excludes:
breath-holding attacks (R06.8)
gender identity disorder of childhood (F64.2)
hypersomnolence and megaphagia (Kleine-Levin syndrome) (G47.8)
obsessive-compulsive disorder (F42.–)
sleep disorders (F51.–)

F98.0 Nonorganic enuresis

A disorder characterized by involuntary voiding of urine, by day and/or by night, which is abnormal in relation to the individual's mental age and which is not a consequence of a lack of bladder control due to any neurological disorder, to epileptic attacks, or to any structural abnormality of the urinary tract. The enuresis may have been present from birth (i.e. an abnormal extension of the normal infantile incontinence) or it may have arisen following a period of acquired bladder control. The later onset (or secondary) variety usually begins about the age of 5 to 7 years. The enuresis may constitute a monosymptomatic condition or it may be associated with a more widespread emotional or behavioural disorder. In the latter case there is uncertainty over the mechanisms involved in the association. Emotional problems may arise as a secondary consequence of the distress or stigma that results from enuresis, the enuresis may form part of some other psychiatric disorder, or both the enuresis and the emotional/behavioural disturbance may arise in parallel from related etiological factors. There is no straightforward, unambiguous way of deciding between these alternatives in the individual case, and the diagnosis should be made on the basis of which type of disturbance (i.e. enuresis or emotional/ behavioural disorder) constitutes the main problem.

Diagnostic guidelines

There is no clear-cut demarcation between an enuresis disorder and the normal variations in the age of acquisition of bladder control. However, enuresis would not ordinarily be diagnosed in a child under the age of 5 years or with a mental age under 4 years. If the enuresis is associated with some (other) emotional or behavioural disorder, enuresis would normally constitute the primary diagnosis only if the involuntary voiding of urine occurred at least several times per week and if the other symptoms showed some temporal covariation with the enuresis. Enuresis sometimes occurs in conjunction with encopresis; when this is the case, encopresis should be diagnosed.

Occasionally, children develop transient enuresis as a result of cystitis or polyuria (as from diabetes). However, these do not constitute a sufficient explanation for enuresis that persists after the infection has been cured or after the polyuria has been brought under control. Not infrequently, the cystitis may be secondary to an enuresis that has arisen by ascending infection up the urinary tract as a result of persistent wetness (especially in girls).

Includes:

enuresis (primary) (secondary) of nonorganic origin
functional or psychogenic enuresis
urinary incontinence of nonorganic origin

Excludes:

enuresis NOS (R32)

A fifth character may be used to provide a more detailed classification of
nonorganic enuresis. The following has been put forward by the
British Paediatric Association.

F98.00   Primary enuresis, unspecified

F98.01   Primary nocturnal enuresis

F98.02   Primary diurnal (and nocturnal) enuresis

F98.03   Secondary enuresis, unspecified

F98.04   Secondary nocturnal enuresis

F98.05   Secondary diurnal (and nocturnal) enuresis

F98.1   Nonorganic encopresis

Repeated voluntary or involuntary passage of faeces, usually of normal or near-normal consistency, in places not appropriate for that purpose in the individual's own sociocultural setting. The condition may represent an abnormal continuation of normal infantile incontinence, it may involve a loss of continence following the acquisition of bowel control, or it may involve the deliberate deposition of faeces in inappropriate places in spite of normal physiological bowel control. The condition may occur as a monosymptomatic disorder, or it may form part of a wider disorder, especially an emotional disorder (F93.–) or a conduct disorder (F91.–).

Diagnostic guidelines

The crucial diagnostic feature is the inappropriate placement of faeces. The condition may arise in several different ways. First, it may represent a lack of adequate toilet-training or of adequate response to training, with the history being one of continuous failure ever to acquire adequate bowel control. Second, it may reflect a psychologically determined disorder in which there is normal physiological control over defecation but, for some reason, a reluctance, resistance, or failure to conform to social norms in defecating in acceptable places. Third, it may stem from physiological retention, involving impaction of faeces, with secondary overflow and deposition of faeces in inappropriate places. Such retention may arise from parent/child battles over bowel-training, from withholding of faeces because of painful defecation (e.g. as a consequence of anal fissure), or for other reasons.

In some instances, the encopresis may be accompanied by smearing of faeces over the body or over the external environment and, less commonly, there may be anal fingering or masturbation. There is usually some degree of associated emotional/behavioural disturbance. There is no clear-cut demarcation between encopresis with associated emotion-

al/behavioural disturbance and some other psychiatric disorder that
includes encopresis as a subsidiary symptom. The recommended guideline is to code encopresis if that is the predominant phenomenon and the
other disorder if it is not (or if the frequency of the encopresis is less than
once a month). Encopresis and enuresis are not infrequently associated
and, when this is the case, the coding of encopresis should have precedence. Encopresis may sometimes follow an organic condition such as
anal fissure or a gastrointestinal infection; the organic condition should
be the sole coding if it constitutes a sufficient explanation for the faecal
soiling but, if it serves as precipitant but not a sufficient cause, encopresis should be coded (in addition to the somatic condition).

Differential diagnosis.
It is important to consider the following:

(a)   encopresis due to organic disease such as aganglionic megacolon
       (Q43.1) or spina bifida (Q05.–) (note, however, that encopresis may
       accompany or follow conditions such as anal fissure or gastrointestinal
       infection);

(b)   constipation involving faecal blockage resulting in 'overflow' faecal
       soiling of liquid or semiliquid faeces (K59.0); if, as happens in some
       cases, encopresis and constipation coexist, encopresis should be coded
       (with an additional code, if appropriate, to identify the cause of the con-
       stipation).

F98.2   *Feeding disorder of infancy and childhood*
A feeding disorder of varying manifestations, usually specific to infancy
and early childhood. It generally involves refusal of food and extreme
faddiness in the presence of an adequate food supply and a reasonably
competent care-giver, and the absence of organic disease. There may or
may not be associated rumination (repeated regurgitation without nausea
or gastrointestinal illness).

Diagnostic guidelines
Minor difficulties in eating are very common in infancy and childhood
(in the form of faddiness, supposed undereating, or supposed overeating). In themselves, these should not be considered as indicative of disorder. Disorder should be diagnosed only if the difficulties are clearly
beyond the normal range, if the nature of the eating problem is qualitatively abnormal in character, or if the child fails to gain weight or loses
weight over a period of at least 1 month.

Includes:
rumination disorder of infancy

Differential diagnosis
It is important to differentiate this disorder from:

(a)   conditions where the child readily takes food from adults other than the usual care-giver;
(b)   organic disease sufficient to explain the food refusal;
(c)   anorexia nervosa and other eating disorders (F50.–);
(d)   broader psychiatric disorder;
(e)   pica (F98.3);
(f)   feeding difficulties and mismanagement (R63.3).

F98.3   *Pica of infancy and childhood*
Persistent eating of non-nutritive substances (soil, paint chippings, etc). Pica may occur as one of many symptoms of a more widespread psychiatric disorder (such as autism), or as a relatively isolated psychopathological behaviour; *only* in the latter case should this code be used. The phenomenon is most common in mentally retarded children; if mental retardation is also present, it should be coded (F70–79). However, pica may also occur in children (usually young children) of normal intelligence.

F98.4   *Stereotyped movement disorders*
Voluntary, repetitive, stereotyped, nonfunctional (and often rhythmic) movements that do not form part of any recognized psychiatric or neurological condition. When such movements occur as symptoms of some other disorder, only the overall disorder should be coded (i.e. F98.4 should not be used). The movements that are noninjurious include: body-rocking, head-rocking, hair-plucking, hair-twisting, finger-flicking mannerisms, and hand-flapping. (Nail-biting, thumb-sucking, and nose-picking should not be included as they are not good indicators of psychopathology, and are not of sufficient public health importance to warrant classification.) Stereotyped self-injurious behaviour includes repetitive head-banging, face-slapping, eye-poking, and biting of hands, lips or other body parts. All the stereotyped movement disorders occur most frequently in association with mental retardation; when this is the case, *both* disorders should be coded.

Eye-poking is particularly common in children with visual impairment. However, the visual disability does not constitute a sufficient explanation, and when both eye-poking and blindness (or partial blind-ness) occur, both should be coded: eye-poking under F98.4 and the visu-al condition under the appropriate somatic disorder code.

Excludes:
abnormal involuntary movements (R25.–)
movement disorders of organic origin (G20–G26)
nail-biting, nose-picking, thumb-sucking (F98.8)
obsessive-compulsive disorder (F42.–)
stereotypies that are part of a broader psychiatric condition (such as per-vasive developmental disorder)
tic disorders (F95.–)
trichotillomania (F63.3)

F98.5   *Stuttering [stammering]*
Speech that is characterized by frequent repetition or prolongation of sounds or syllables or words, or by frequent hesitations or pauses that disrupt the rhythmic flow of speech. Minor dysrhythmias of this type are quite common as a transient phase in early childhood, or as a minor but persistent speech feature in later childhood and adult life. They should be classified as a disorder only if their severity is such as markedly to disturb the fluency of speech. There may be associated movements of the face and/or other parts of the body that coincide in time with the rep-etitions, prolongations, or pauses in speech flow. Stuttering should be differentiated from cluttering (see below) and from tics. In some cases there may be an associated developmental disorder of speech or lan-guage, in which case this should be separately coded under F80.–.

Excludes:
cluttering (F98.6)
neurological disorder giving rise to speech dysrhythmias (Chapter VI of ICD–10)
obsessive-compulsive disorder (F42.–)
tic disorders (F95.–)

F98.6   *Cluttering*
A rapid rate of speech with breakdown in fluency, but no repetitions or hesitations, of a severity to give rise to reduced speech intelligibility. Speech is erratic and dysrhythmic, with rapid, jerky spurts that usually involve faulty phrasing patterns (e.g. alternating pauses and bursts of

speech, producing groups of words unrelated to the grammatical structure of the sentence).

Excludes:
neurological disorder giving rise to speech dysrhythmias (Chapter VI of
    ICD–10)
obsessive-compulsive disorder (F42.–)
stuttering (F98.5)
tic disorders (F95.–)

F98.8   ***Other specified behavioural and emotional disorders with onset usually occurring in childhood and adolescence***

Includes:
attention deficit disorder without hyperactivity
(excessive) masturbation
nail-biting
nose-picking
thumb-sucking

F98.9   ***Unspecified behavioural and emotional disorders with onset usually
occurring in childhood and adolescence***

F99 is a residual category for the whole of Axis One, and not just for the
block on behavioural and emotional disorders with onset usually occurring in childhood and adolescence. It is therefore placed right at the end
of the axis and not here.

F00-F09	Organic, including symptomatic, mental disorders
F00	Dementia in Alzheimer's disease
F01	Vascular dementia
F02	Dementia in other diseases classified elsewhere
F03	Dementia, unspecified
F04	Organic amnesic syndrome, other than induced by alcohol or other psychoactive substances
F05	Delerium, other than induced by alcohol and other psychoactive substances
F06	Other mental disorders due to brain damage or dysfunction or to physical disease
F07	Personality and behavioural disorders due to brain disease, damage or dysfunction
F09	Unspecified organic or symptomatic mental disorder

A syndrome of prominent impairment of recent and remote memory while immediate recall is preserved, with reduced ability to learn new material and disorientation in time. Confabulation may be a marked feature, but perception and other cognitive functions, including the intellect, are usually intact. The prognosis depends on the course of the underlying lesion.

Includes:
Korsakov's psychosis or syndrome, nonalcoholic

Excludes:
amnesia: NOS (R41.3)
         anterograde (R41.1)
         dissociative (44.0)
         retrograde (41.1)
Korsakov's syndrome: alcohol-induced or unspecified (10.6)
                induced by other psychoactive substances
                (11 –19 with common fourth character.6)

F05   Delirium, other than induced by alcohol and other psychoactive substances

An etiologically nonspecific organic cerebral syndrome characterized by concurrent disturbances of consciousness and attention, perception,

thinking, memory, psychomotor behaviour, emotion, and the sleep
–wake schedule. The duration is variable and the degree of severity
ranges from mild to very severe.

Includes:
acute or subacute: brain syndrome
                   confusional state (non-alcoholic)
                   infective psychosis
                   organic reaction
                   psycho-organic syndrome

Excludes:
                   delirium tremens, alcohol-induced or unspecified
                   (10.4)

F06   Other mental disorders due to brain damage or dysfunction or to physical disease

Includes miscellaneous conditions causally related to brain disorder due
to primary cerebral disease, to systemic disease affecting the brain sec-
ondarily, to exogenous toxic substances or hormones, to endocrine disorders, or to other somatic illnesses.

Excludes:
disorders associated with:
delirium (05. –)
dementia as classified in 00 –09
resulting from use of alcohol and other psychoactive substances (10 –19)

F07   Personality and behavioural disorders due to brain disease, damage or dysfunction

Alteration of personality and behaviour can be a residual or concomitant
disorder of brain disease, damage or dysfunction.

F09   Unspecified organic or symptomatic mental disorder

Includes:
Psychosis: Organic NOS
           symptomatic NOS

Excludes:
           psychosis NOS (F29)

F10–F19   **Mental and behavioural disorders due to psychoactive substance use**

F10   **Mental and behavioural disorders due to use of alcohol**

F11   **Mental and behavioural disorders due to use of opiods**

F12   **Mental and behavioural disorders due to use of cannabinoids**

F13   **Mental and behavioural disorders due to use of sedatives or hypnotics**

F14   **Mental and behavioural disorders due to use of cocaine**

F15   **Mental and behavioural disorders due to use of other stimulants, including caffeine**

F16   **Mental and behavioural disorders due to use of hallucingoens**

F17   **Mental and behavioural disorders due to use of tobacco**

F18   **Mental and behavioural disorders due to use of volatile solvents**

F19   **Mental and behavioural disorders due to multiple drug use and use of other psychoactive substances**

This section contains a wide variety of disorders that differ in severity and clinical form but that are attributable to the use of one or more psychoactive substances, which may or may not have been medically prescribed. The third character of the code identifies the substance involved, and the fourth character specifies the clinical state. The codes should be used, as required, for each substance specified, but it should be noted that not all fourth-character codes are applicable to all substances.

Identification of the psychoactive substance should be based on as many sources of information as possible. These include self-report data, analysis and blood or other body fluids, characteristic physical and psychological symptoms, clinical signs and behaviour, and other evidence such as a drug being in the patient's possession or reports from informed third parties. Many drug users take more than one type of psychoactive substance. The principal diagnosis should be classified, whenever possible, according to the substance or class of substances that has caused or contributed most to the presenting clinical syndrome. Subsidiary diagnoses should be coded when other psychoactive substances have been taken in intoxicating amounts (common fourth character .0) or to the extent of causing harm (common fourth character .1), dependence (common fourth character .2) or other disorders (common fourth character .3–.9).

Only in cases in which patterns of drug taking are chaotic and indiscriminate, or in which the contributions of different drugs are inextricably mixed, should the diagnosis of disorders resulting from multiple drug use (F19) be coded.

Excludes: abuse of non-dependence-producing substances (F55)

The following fourth-character subdivisions are for use with categories (F10–F19)

.0   Acute intoxication
A condition that follows the administration of a psychoactive substance resulting in disturbances in level of consciousness, cognition, perception, affect or behaviour, or other psychophysiological functions and responses. The disturbances are directly related to the acute pharmacological effects of the substance and resolve with time, with complete recovery, except where tissue damage or other complications have arisen. Complications may include trauma, inhalation of vomitus, delirium, coma, convulsions, and other medical complications. The nature of these complications depends on the pharmacological class of substance and mode of administration.

Acute drunkenness in alcoholism
'Bad trips' (drugs)
Drunkenness NOS
Pathological intoxication
Trance and possession disorders in psychoactive substances intoxication

.1   Harmful use
A pattern of psychoactive substance use that is causing damage to health. The damage may be physical (as in cases of hepatitis from the self-administration of injected psychoactive substances) or mental (e.g. episodes of depressive disorder secondary to heavy consumption of alcohol).

Psychoactive substance abuse

.2   Dependence syndrome
A cluster of behavioural, cognitive, and physiological phenomena that develop after repeated substance use and that typically include a strong desire to take the drug, difficulties in controlling its use, persisting in its use despite harmful consequences, a higher priority given to drug use than to other activities and obligations, increased tolerance, and sometimes a physical withdrawal state.

The dependence syndrome may be present for a specific psychoactive substance (e.g. tobacco, alcohol, or diazepam), for a class of substances (e.g. opioid drugs), or for a wider range of pharmacologically different psychoactive substances.

Chronic alcoholism
Dipsomania
Drug addiction

.3 Withdrawal state

A group of symptoms of variable clustering and severity occurring on absolute or relative withdrawal of a substance after persistent use of that substance. The onset and course of the withdrawal state are time-limited and are related to the type of substance and dose being used immediately before cessation or reduction of use. The withdrawal state may be complicated by convulsions.

.4 Withdrawal state with delirium

A condition where the withdrawal state as defined in 19.3 is complicated by delirium as defined in 05. Convulsions may also occur. When organic factors are also considered to play a role in the etiology, the condition should be classified to 05.8.

Includes: Delirium tremens, alcohol-related

.5 Psychotic disorder

A cluster of psychotic phenomena that occur during or following substance use but that are not explained on the basis of acute intoxication alone and do not form part of a withdrawal state. The disorder is characterized by hallucinations (typically auditory, but often in more than one sensory modality), perceptual distortions, delusions (often of a paranoid or persecutory nature), psychomotor disturbances (excitement or stupor), and an abnormal affect, which may range from intense fear to ecstasy. The sensorium is usually clear but some degree of clouding of consciousness, though not severe confusion, may be present.

Includes: alcoholic:
       hallucinosis
       jealousy
       paranoia
       psychosis NOS

One

Excludes: alcohol- or other psychoactive substance-induced residual and late-onset psychotic disorder (10–19 with common fourth character.7)

.6   Amnesic syndrome

A syndrome associated with chronic prominent impairment of recent and remote memory. Immediate recall is usually preserved. Recent memory is characteristically more disturbed than remote memory. Disturbances of time sense and ordering of events are usually evident, as are difficulties in learning new material. Confabulation may be marked but is not invariably present. Other cognitive functions are usually relatively well preserved and amnesic defects are out of proportion to other disturbances.

Includes: amnestic disorder, alcohol or drug-induced
Korsakov's psychosis or syndrome, alcohol-, or other
psychoactive substance-induced or unspecified

Excludes: nonalcoholic Korsakov's syndrome (04)

.7   Residual and late-onset psychotic disorder

A disorder in which alcohol- or psychoactive substance-induced changes of cognition, affect, personality, or behaviour persist beyond the period during which a direct psychoactive substance-related effect might reasonably be assumed to be operating. Onset of the disorder should be directly related to the use of the substance. Cases in which initial onset of the state occurs later than episode(s) of such substance use should be coded here only where clear and strong evidence is available to attribute the state to the residual effect of the psychoactive substance. Flashbacks may be distinguished from psychotic state partly by their episodic nature, frequently of very short duration and by their duplication of previous alcohol or other psychoactive substance-related experiences.

Includes: alcoholic dementia NOS
chronic alcoholic brain syndrome
dementia and other milder forms of persisting impairment of
  cognitive functions
flashbacks
late-onset psychoactive substance-induced psychotic disorder
post hallucinogen perception disorder
residual:
  affective disorder
  disorder of personality and behaviour

Excludes: alcohol- or psychoactive substance-induced:
> Korsakov's syndrome (10–19 with common fourth character)
> psychotic state (10–19 with common fourth character .5)

.8   *Other mental and behavioural disorders*

.9   *Unspecified mental and behavioural disorder*
The above digits should be used with the categories listed below
(F10–F19)

F10   Mental and behavioural disorders due to use of alcohol

F11   Mental and behavioural disorders due to use of opioids

F12   Mental and behavioural disorders due to use of cannabinoids

**F13   Mental and behavioural disorders due to use of sedatives or
hypnotics**

F14   Mental and behavioural disorders due to use of cocaine

**F15   Mental and behavioural disorders due to use of other stimulants,
including caffeine**

F16   Mental and behavioural disorders due to use of hallucinogens

F17   Mental and behavioural disorders due to use of tobacco

F18   Mental and behavioural disorders due to use of volatile solvents

**F19   Mental and behavioural disorders due to multiple drug use and
use of other psychoactive substances**

This category should be used when two or more substances are known to
be involved, but it is impossible to assess which substance is contribut-
ing most to the disorders. It should also be used when the exact identity
of some or even all the substances being used is uncertain or unknown,
since many multiple drug users themselves often do not know the details
of what they are taking.

Includes: misuse of drugs NOS

F20–F29   **Schizophrenia, schizotypal and delusional disorders**

F20   Schizophrenia

    F20.0   Paranoid schizophrenia

    F20.1   Hebephrenic schizophrenia

    F20.2   Catatonic schizophrenia

    F20.3   Undifferentiated schizophrenia

    F20.4   Post-schizophrenic depression

    F20.5   Residual schizophrenia

    F20.6   Simple schizophrenia

    F20.8   Other schizophrenia

    F20.9   Schizophrenia, unspecified

    A fifth character may be used to classify course:

    F20.x0   Continuous

    F20.x1   Episodic with progressive deficit

    F20.x2   Episodic with stable deficit

    F20.x3   Episodic remittent

    F20.x4   Incomplete remission

    F20.x5   Complete remission

    F20.x8   Other

    F20.x9   Course uncertain, period of observation too short

F21   Schizotypal disorder

F22   Persistent delusional disorders

    F22.0   Delusional disorder

    F22.8   Other persistent delusional disorders

    F22.9   Persistent delusional disorder, unspecified

F23   Acute and transient psychotic disorders

    F23.0   Acute polymorphic psychotic disorder without symptoms of schizophrenia

    F23.1   Acute polymorphic psychotic disorder with symptoms of schizophrenia

    F23.2   Acute schizophrenia-like psychotic disorder

    F23.3   Other acute predominantly delusional psychotic disorder

    F23.8   Other acute and transient psychotic disorders

    F23.9   Acute and transient psychotic disorder, unspecified

    A fifth character may be used to identify the presence or absence of associated acute stress:

F23.x0   Without associated acute stress
F23.x1   With associated acute stress

F24   Induced delusional disorder

F25   Schizoaffective disorders
F25.0   Schizoaffective disorder, manic type
F25.1   Schizoaffective disorder, depressive type
F25.2   Schizoaffective disorder, mixed type
F25.8   Other schizoaffective disorders
F25.9   Schizoaffective disorder, unspecified

F28   Other nonorganic psychotic disorders

F29   Unspecified nonorganic psychosis

Introduction

Schizophrenia is the commonest and most important disorder of this group. Schizotypal disorder possesses many of the characteristic features of schizophrenic disorders and is probably genetically related to them; however, the hallucinations, delusions, and gross behavioural disturbances of schizophrenia itself are absent and so this disorder does not always come to medical attention. Most of the delusional disorders are probably unrelated to schizophrenia, although they may be difficult to distinguish clinically, particularly in their early stages. They form a heterogeneous and poorly understood collection of disorders, which can conveniently be divided according to their typical duration into a group of persistent delusional disorders and a larger group of acute and transient psychotic disorders. The latter appear to be particularly common in developing countries. The subdivisions listed here should be regarded as provisional. Schizoaffective disorders have been retained in this section in spite of their controversial nature.

F20   Schizophrenia

The schizophrenic disorders are characterized in general by fundamental and characteristic distortions of thinking and perception, and by inappropriate or blunted affect. Clear consciousness and intellectual capacity are usually maintained, although certain cognitive deficits may evolve in the course of time. The disturbance involves the most basic functions that give the normal person a feeling of individuality, uniqueness, and self-direction. The most intimate thoughts, feelings, and acts are often felt to be known to or shared by others, and explanatory delusions may develop, to the effect that natural or supernatural forces are at work to influence the afflicted individual's thoughts and actions in ways that are often bizarre. The individual may see himself or herself as the pivot of all that happens. Hallucinations, especially auditory, are common and may comment on the individual's behaviour or thoughts. Perception is frequently disturbed in other ways: colours or sounds may seem unduly vivid or altered in quality, and irrelevant features of ordinary things may appear more important than the whole object or situation. Perplexity is also common early on and frequently leads to a belief that everyday situations possess a special, usually sinister, meaning intended uniquely for the individual. In the characteristic schizo-phrenic disturbance of thinking, peripheral and irrelevant features of a total concept, which are inhibited in normal directed mental activity, are brought to the fore and utilized in place of those that are relevant and appropriate to the situation. Thus thinking becomes vague, elliptical, and obscure, and its expression in speech sometimes incomprehensible. Breaks and interpolations in the train of thought are frequent, and thoughts may seem to be withdrawn by some outside agency. Mood is characteristically shallow, capricious, or incongruous. Ambivalence and disturbance of volition may appear as inertia, negativism, or stupor. Catatonia may be present. The onset may be acute, with seriously disturbed behaviour, or insidious, with a gradual development of odd ideas and conduct. The course of the disorder shows equally great variation and is by no means inevitably chronic or deteriorating (the course is specified by five-character categories). In a proportion of cases, which may vary in different cultures and populations, the outcome is complete, or nearly complete, recovery. The sexes are approximately equally affected but the onset tends to be later in women.

Although no strictly pathognomonic symptoms can be identified, for practical purposes it is useful to divide the above symptoms into groups that have special importance for the diagnosis and often occur together, such as:

(a) thought echo, thought insertion or withdrawal, and thought broadcasting;

(b) delusions of control, influence, or passivity, clearly referred to body or limb movements or specific thoughts, actions, or sensations; delusional perception;

(c) hallucinatory voices giving a running commentary on the patient's behaviour, or discussing the patient among themselves, or other types of hallucinatory voices coming from some part of the body;

(d)   persistent delusions of other kinds that are culturally inappropriate and completely impossible, such as religious or political identity, or super-human powers and abilities (e.g. being able to control the weather, or being in communication with aliens from another world);

(e)   persistent hallucinations in any modality, when accompanied either by fleeting or half-formed delusions without clear affective content, or by persistent over-valued ideas, or when occurring every day for weeks or months on end;

(f)   breaks or interpolations in the train of thought, resulting in incoherence or irrelevant speech, or neologisms;

(g)   catatonic behaviour, such as excitement, posturing, or waxy flexibility, negativism, mutism, and stupor;

(h)   'negative' symptoms such as marked apathy, paucity of speech, and blunting or incongruity of emotional responses, usually resulting in social withdrawal and lowering of social performance; it must be clear that these are not due to depression or to neuroleptic medication;

(i)   a significant and consistent change in the overall quality of some aspects of personal behaviour, manifest as loss of interest, aimlessness, idleness, a self-absorbed attitude, and social withdrawal.

Diagnostic guidelines

The normal requirement for a diagnosis of schizophrenia is that a minimum of one very clear symptom (and usually two or more if less clear-cut) belonging to any one of the groups listed as (a) to (d) above, or symptoms from at least two of the groups referred to as (e) to (h), should have been clearly present for most of the time *during a period of 1 month or more*. Conditions meeting such symptomatic requirements but of duration less than 1 month (whether treated or not) should be diagnosed in the first instance as acute schizophrenia-like psychotic disorder (F23.2) and reclassified as schizophrenia if the symptoms persist for longer periods. Symptom (i) in the above list applies only to a diagnosis of Simple Schizophrenia (F20.6), and a duration of at least one year is required.

Viewed retrospectively, it may be clear that a prodromal phase in which symptoms and behaviour, such as loss of interest in work, social activities, and personal appearance and hygiene, together with generalized anxiety and mild degrees of depression and preoccupation, preceded the onset of psychotic symptoms by weeks or even months. Because of the difficulty in timing onset, the 1-month duration criterion applies only to the specific symptoms listed above and not to any prodromal nonpsychotic phase.

One

The diagnosis of schizophrenia should not be made in the presence of extensive depressive or manic symptoms unless it is clear that schizophrenic symptoms antedated the affective disturbance. If both schizophrenic and affective symptoms develop together and are evenly balanced, the diagnosis of schizoaffective disorder (F25.–) should be made, even if the schizophrenic symptoms by themselves would have justified the diagnosis of schizophrenia. Schizophrenia should not be diagnosed in the presence of overt brain disease or during states of drug intoxication or withdrawal. Similar disorders developing in the presence of epilepsy or other brain disease should be coded under F06.2 and those induced by drugs under F1x.5.

Pattern of course
The course of schizophrenic disorders can be classified by using the following five-character codes:

F20.x0 Continuous
F20.x1 Episodic with progressive deficit
F20.x2 Episodic with stable deficit
F20.x3 Episodic remittent
F20.x4 Incomplete remission
F20.x5 Complete remission
F20.x8 Other
F20.x9 Course uncertain, period of observation too short

F20.0   Paranoid schizophrenia
This is the commonest type of schizophrenia in most parts of the world. The clinical picture is dominated by relatively stable, often paranoid, delusions, usually accompanied by hallucinations, particularly of the auditory variety, and perceptual disturbances. Disturbances of affect, volition, and speech, and catatonic symptoms, are not prominent.

Examples of the most common paranoid symptoms are:

(a) delusions of persecution, reference, exalted birth, special mission, bodily change, or jealousy;
(b) hallucinatory voices that threaten the patient or give commands, or auditory hallucinations without verbal form, such as whistling, humming, or laughing;
(c) hallucinations of smell or taste, or of sexual or other bodily sensations; visual hallucinations may occur but are rarely predominant.

Thought disorder may be obvious in acute states, but if so it does not prevent the typical delusions or hallucinations from being described clearly. Affect is usually less blunted than in other varieties of schizophrenia, but a minor degree of incongruity is common, as are mood disturbances such as irritability, sudden anger, fearfulness, and suspicion. 'Negative' symptoms such as blunting of affect and impaired volition are often present but do not dominate the clinical picture.

The course of paranoid schizophrenia may be episodic, with partial or complete remissions, or chronic. In chronic cases, the florid symptoms persist over years and it is difficult to distinguish discrete episodes. The onset tends to be later than in the hebephrenic and catatonic forms.

Diagnostic guidelines
The general criteria for a diagnosis of schizophrenia (see introduction to F20 above) must be satisfied. In addition, hallucinations and/or delusions must be prominent, and disturbances of affect, volition and speech, and catatonic symptoms must be relatively inconspicuous. The hallucinations will usually be of the kind described in (b) and (c) above. Delusions can be of almost any kind but delusions of control, influence, or passivity, and persecutory beliefs of various kinds are the most characteristic.

Includes: paraphrenic schizophrenia

Differential diagnosis.
It is important to exclude epileptic and drug-induced psychoses, and to remember that persecutory delusions might carry little diagnostic weight in people from certain countries or cultures.

Excludes: involutional paranoid state (F22.8)
            paranoia (F22.0)

F20.1   Hebephrenic schizophrenia
A form of schizophrenia in which affective changes are prominent, delusions and hallucinations fleeting and fragmentary, behaviour irresponsible and unpredictable, and mannerisms common. The mood is shallow and inappropriate and often accompanied by giggling or self-satisfied, self-absorbed smiling, or by a lofty manner, grimaces, mannerisms, pranks, hypochondriacal complaints, and reiterated phrases. Thought is disorganized and speech rambling and incoherent. There is a tendency to remain solitary, and behaviour seems empty of purpose and feeling. This form of schizophrenia usually starts between the ages of 15 and 25 years

and tends to have a poor prognosis because of the rapid development of 'negative' symptoms, particularly flattening of affect and loss of volition.

In addition, disturbances of affect and volition, and thought disorder are usually prominent. Hallucinations and delusions may be present but are not usually prominent. Drive and determination are lost and goals abandoned, so that the patient's behaviour becomes characteristically aimless and empty of purpose. A superficial and manneristic preoccupation with religion, philosophy, and other abstract themes may add to the listener's difficulty in following the train of thought.

Diagnostic guidelines

The general criteria for a diagnosis of schizophrenia (see introduction to F20 above) must be satisfied. Hebephrenia should normally be diagnosed for the first time only in adolescents or young adults. The premorbid personality is characteristically, but not necessarily, rather shy and solitary. For a confident diagnosis of hebephrenia, a period of 2 or 3 months of continuous observation is usually necessary, in order to ensure that the characteristic behaviours described above are sustained.

Includes: disorganized schizophrenia
         hebephrenia

F20.2   Catatonic schizophrenia

Prominent psychomotor disturbances are essential and dominant features and may alternate between extremes such as hyperkinesis and stupor, or automatic obedience and negativism. Constrained attitudes and postures may be maintained for long periods. Episodes of violent excitement may be a striking feature of the condition.

For reasons that are poorly understood, catatonic schizophrenia is now rarely seen in industrial countries, though it remains common elsewhere. These catatonic phenomena may be combined with a dream-like (oneiroid) state with vivid scenic hallucinations.

Diagnostic guidelines

The general criteria for a diagnosis of schizophrenia (see introduction to F20 above) must be satisfied. Transitory and isolated catatonic symptoms may occur in the context of any other subtype of schizophrenia, but for a diagnosis of catatonic schizophrenia one or more of the following behaviours should dominate the clinical picture:

(a) stupor (marked decrease in reactivity to the environment and in spontaneous movements and activity) or mutism;

(b) excitement (apparently purposeless motor activity, not influenced by external stimuli);

(c) posturing (voluntary assumption and maintenance of inappropriate or bizarre postures);

(d) negativism (an apparently motiveless resistance to all instructions or attempts to be moved, or movement in the opposite direction);

(e) rigidity (maintenance of a rigid posture against efforts to be moved);

(f) waxy flexibility (maintenance of limbs and body in externally imposed positions); and

(g) other symptoms such as command automatism (automatic compliance with instructions), and perseveration of words and phrases.

In uncommunicative patients with behavioural manifestations of catatonic disorder, the diagnosis of schizophrenia may have to be provisional until adequate evidence of the presence of other symptoms is obtained. It is also vital to appreciate that catatonic symptoms are not diagnostic of schizophrenia. A catatonic symptom or symptoms may also be provoked by brain disease, metabolic disturbances, or alcohol and drugs, and may also occur in mood disorders.

Includes: catatonic stupor
schizophrenic catalepsy
schizophrenic catatonia
schizophrenic flexibilitas cerea

F20.3 *Undifferentiated schizophrenia*
Conditions meeting the general diagnostic criteria for schizophrenia (see introduction to F20 above) but not conforming to any of the above subtypes (F20.0–F20.2), or exhibiting the features of more than one of them without a clear predominance of a particular set of diagnostic characteristics. This rubric should be used only for psychotic conditions (i.e. residual schizophrenia, F20.5, and post-schizophrenic depression, F20.4, are excluded) and after an attempt has been made to classify the condition into one of the three preceding categories.

Diagnostic guidelines
This category should be reserved for disorders that:

(a) meet the general criteria for schizophrenia;

(b) either without sufficient symptoms to meet the criteria for only one of the subtypes F20.0, F20.1, F20.2, F20.4, or F20.5, or with so many symptoms that the criteria for more than one of the paranoid (F20.0), hebephrenic (F20.1), or catatonic (F20.2) subtypes are met.

Includes: atypical schizophrenia

F20.4 Post-schizophrenic depression

A depressive episode, which may be prolonged, arising in the aftermath of a schizophrenic illness. Some schizophrenic symptoms must still be present but no longer dominate the clinical picture. These persisting schizophrenic symptoms may be 'positive' or 'negative', though the latter are more common. It is uncertain, and immaterial to the diagnosis, to what extent the depressive symptoms have merely been uncovered by the resolution of earlier psychotic symptoms (rather than being a new development) or are an intrinsic part of schizophrenia rather than a psychological reaction to it. They are rarely sufficiently severe or extensive to meet criteria for a severe depressive episode (F32.2 and F32.3), and it is often difficult to decide which of the patient's symptoms are due to depression and which to neuroleptic medication or to the impaired volition and affective flattening of schizophrenia itself. This depressive disorder is associated with an increased risk of suicide.

Diagnostic guidelines

The diagnosis should be made only if:

(a) the patient has had a schizophrenic illness meeting the general criteria for schizophrenia (see introduction to F20 above) within the past 12 months;

(b) some schizophrenic symptoms are still present; and

(c) the depressive symptoms are prominent and distressing, fulfilling at least the criteria for a depressive episode (F32.–), and have been present for at least 2 weeks.

If the patient no longer has any schizophrenic symptoms, a depressive episode should be diagnosed (F32.–). If schizophrenic symptoms are still florid and prominent, the diagnosis should remain that of the appropriate schizophrenic subtype (F20.0, F20.1, F20.2, or F20.3).

F20.5 Residual schizophrenia

A chronic stage in the development of a schizophrenic disorder in which there has been a clear progression from an early stage (comprising one or more episodes with psychotic symptoms meeting the general criteria for schizophrenia described above) to a later stage characterized by long-term, though not necessarily irreversible, 'negative' symptoms.

Diagnostic guidelines
For a confident diagnosis, the following requirements should be met:

(a) prominent 'negative' schizophrenic symptoms, i.e. psychomotor slowing, underactivity, blunting of affect, passivity and lack of initiative, poverty of quantity or content of speech, poor nonverbal communication by facial expression, eye contact, voice modulation, and posture, poor self-care and social performance;

(b) evidence in the past of at least one clear-cut psychotic episode meeting the diagnostic criteria for schizophrenia;

(c) a period of *at least 1 year* during which the intensity and frequency of florid symptoms such as delusions and hallucinations have been minimal or substantially reduced *and* the 'negative' schizophrenic syndrome has been present;

(d) absence of dementia or other organic brain disease or disorder, and of chronic depression or institutionalism sufficient to explain the negative impairments.

If adequate information about the patient's previous history cannot be obtained, and it therefore cannot be established that criteria for schizophrenia have been met at some time in the past, it may be necessary to make a provisional diagnosis of residual schizophrenia.

Includes: chronic undifferentiated schizophrenia
        'Restzustand'
        schizophrenic residual state

F20.6   Simple schizophrenia

An uncommon disorder in which there is an insidious but progressive development of oddities of conduct, inability to meet the demands of society, and decline in total performance. Delusions and hallucinations are not evident, and the disorder is less obviously psychotic than the hebephrenic, paranoid, and catatonic subtypes of schizophrenia. The characteristic "negative" features of residual schizophrenia (e.g. blunting of affect, loss of volition) develop without being preceded by any overt psychotic symptoms. With increasing social impoverishment, vagrancy may ensue and the individual may then become self-absorbed, idle, and aimless.

Diagnostic guidelines

Simple schizophrenia is a difficult diagnosis to make with any confidence because it depends on establishing the slowly progressive development of the characteristic 'negative' symptoms of residual schizophrenia (see F20.5 above) without any history of hallucinations, delusions, or other manifestations of an earlier psychotic episode, and with significant changes in personal behaviour, manifest as a marked loss of interest, idleness, and social withdrawal over a period of at least one year.

Includes: schizophrenia simplex

F20.8 *Other schizophrenia*

Includes: cenesthopathic schizophrenia

schizophreniform disorder NOS

Excludes: acute schizophrenia-like disorder (F23.2)

cyclic schizophrenia (F25.2)

latent schizophrenia (F23.2)

F20.9 *Schizophrenia, unspecified*

F21 Schizotypal disorder

A disorder characterized by eccentric behaviour and anomalies of thinking and affect which resemble those seen in schizophrenia, though no definite and characteristic schizophrenic anomalies have occurred at any stage. There is no dominant or typical disturbance, but any of the following may be present:

(a) inappropriate or constricted affect (the individual appears cold and aloof);

(b) behaviour or appearance that is odd, eccentric, or peculiar;

(c) poor rapport with others and a tendency to social withdrawal;

(d) odd beliefs or magical thinking, influencing behaviour and inconsistent with subcultural norms;

(e) suspiciousness or paranoid ideas;

(f) obsessive ruminations without inner resistance, often with dysmorphophobic, sexual or aggressive contents;

(g) unusual perceptual experiences including somatosensory (bodily) or other illusions, depersonalization or derealization;

(h) vague, circumstantial, metaphorical, overelaborate, or stereotyped thinking, manifested by odd speech or in other ways, without gross incoherence;

(i)   occasional transient quasi-psychotic episodes with intense illusions, auditory or other hallucinations, and delusion-like ideas, usually occurring without external provocation.

The disorder runs a chronic course with fluctuations of intensity. Occasionally it evolves into overt schizophrenia. There is no definite onset and its evolution and course are usually those of a personality disorder. It is more common in individuals related to schizophrenics and is believed to be part of the genetic 'spectrum' of schizophrenia.

Diagnostic guidelines

This diagnostic rubric is not recommended for general use because it is not clearly demarcated either from simple schizophrenia or from schizoid or paranoid personality disorders. If the term is used, three or four of the typical features listed above should have been present, continuously or episodically, for *at least 2 years*. The individual must never have met criteria for schizophrenia itself. A history of schizophrenia in a first-degree relative gives additional weight to the diagnosis but is not a prerequisite.

Includes: borderline schizophrenia
         latent schizophrenia
         latent schizophrenic reaction
         prepsychotic schizophrenia
         prodromal schizophrenia
         pseudoneurotic schizophrenia
         pseudopsychopathic schizophrenia
         schizotypal personality disorder

Excludes: Asperger's syndrome (F84.5)
         schizoid personality disorder (F60.1)

F22   Persistent delusional disorders

This group includes a variety of disorders in which long-standing delusions constitute the only, or the most conspicuous, clinical characteristic and which cannot be classified as organic, schizophrenic, or affective. They are probably heterogeneous, and have uncertain relationships to schizophrenia. The relative importance of genetic factors, personality characteristics, and life circumstances in their genesis is uncertain and probably variable.

One

F22.0 *Delusional disorder*

This group of disorders is characterized by the development either of a single delusion or of a set of related delusions, which are usually persistent and sometimes lifelong. The delusions are highly variable in content. Often they are persecutory, hypochondriacal, or grandiose, but they may be concerned with litigation or jealousy, or express a conviction that the individual's body is misshapen, or that others think that he or she smells or is homosexual. Other psychopathology is characteristically absent, but depressive symptoms may be present intermittently, and olfactory and tactile hallucinations may develop in some cases. Clear and persistent auditory hallucinations (voices), schizophrenic symptoms such as delusions of control and marked blunting of affect, and definite evidence of brain disease are all incompatible with this diagnosis. However, occasional or transitory auditory hallucinations do not rule out this diagnosis, provided that they are not typically schizophrenic and form only a small part of the overall clinical picture. Although onset is commonly in middle age, sometimes, particularly in the case of beliefs about having a misshapen body, in early adult life or even adolescence. The content of the delusion, and the timing of its emergence, can often be related to the individual's life situation, e.g. persecutory delusions in members of minorities. Apart from actions and attitudes directly related to the delusion or delusional system, affect, speech, and behaviour are normal.

Diagnostic guidelines

Delusions constitute the most conspicuous or the only clinical characteristic. They must be present for at least 3 months and be clearly personal rather than subcultural. Depressive symptoms or even a full-blown depressive episode (F32.–) may be present intermittently, provided that the delusions persist at times when there is no disturbance of mood. There must be no evidence of brain disease, no or only occasional auditory hallucinations, and no history of schizophrenic symptoms (delusions of control, thought broadcasting, etc.).

Includes: paranoia
paranoid psychosis
paranoid state
paraphrenia (late)
sensitiver Beziehungswahn

Excludes: paranoid personality disorder (F60.0)
psychogenic paranoid psychosis (F23.3)

paranoid reaction (F23.3)
paranoid schizophrenia (F20.0)

F22.8 *Other persistent delusional disorders*

This is a residual category for persistent delusional disorders that do not meet the criteria for delusional disorder (F22.0). Disorders in which delusions are accompanied by persistent hallucinatory voices or by schizophrenic symptoms that are insufficient to meet criteria for schizophrenia (F20.–) should be coded here. Delusional disorders that have lasted for less than 3 months should, however, should be coded, at least temporarily, under F23.–.

Includes: delusional dysmorphophobia
             involutional paranoid state
             paranoia querulans

F22.9 *Persistent delusional disorder, unspecified*

F23 **Acute and transient psychotic disorders**

Systematic clinical information that would provide definitive guidance on the classification of acute psychotic disorders is not yet available, and the limited data and clinical tradition that must therefore be used instead do not give rise to concepts that can be clearly defined and separated from each other. In the absence of a tried and tested multi-axial system, the method used here to avoid diagnostic confusion is to construct a diagnostic sequence that reflects the order of priority given to selected key features of the disorder. The order of priority used here is:

(a)   an acute onset (within 2 weeks) as the defining feature of the whole group;
(b)   the presence of typical syndromes;
(c)   the presence of associated acute stress.

The classification is nevertheless arranged so that those who do not agree with this order of priority can still identify acute psychotic disorders with each of these specified features.

It is also recommended that whenever possible a further subdivision of onset be used, if applicable, for all the disorders of this group. *Acute onset* is defined as a change from a state without psychotic features to a clearly abnormal psychotic state, within a period of 2 weeks or less. There is some evidence that acute onset is associated with a good outcome, and it may be that the more abrupt the onset, the better the outcome. It is therefore recommended that, whenever appropriate, *abrupt onset* (within 48 hours or less) be specified.

The *typical syndromes* that have been selected are first, the rapidly changing and variable state, called here 'polymorphic', that has been given prominence in acute psychotic states in several countries, and second, the presence of typical schizophrenic symptoms.

Associated acute stress can also be specified, with a fifth character if desired, in view of its traditional linkage with acute psychosis. The limited evidence available, however, indicates that a substantial proportion of acute psychotic disorders arise without associated stress, and provision has therefore been made for the presence or the absence of stress to be recorded. Associated acute stress is taken to mean that the first psychotic symptoms occur within about 2 weeks of one or more events that would be regarded as stressful to most people in similar circumstances, within the culture of the person concerned. Typical events would be bereavement, unexpected loss of partner or job, marriage, or the psychological trauma of combat, terrorism, and torture. Long-standing difficulties or problems should not be included as a source of stress in this context.

Complete recovery usually occurs within 2 to 3 months, often within a few weeks or even days, and only a small proportion of patients with these disorders develop persistent and disabling states. Unfortunately, the present state of knowledge does not allow the early prediction of that small proportion of patients who will not recover rapidly.

These clinical descriptions and diagnostic guidelines are written on the assumption that they will be used by clinicians who may need to make a diagnosis when having to assess and treat patients within a few days or weeks of the onset of the disorder, not knowing how long the disorder will last. A number of reminders about the time limits and transition from one disorder to another have therefore been included, so as to alert those recording the diagnosis to the need to keep them up to date.

The nomenclature of these acute disorders is as uncertain as their nosological status, but an attempt has been made to use simple and familiar terms. 'Psychotic disorder' is used as a term of convenience for all the members of this group (psychotic is defined in the general introduction, page ?) with an additional qualifying term indicating the major defining feature of each separate type as it appears in the sequence noted above.

Diagnostic guidelines
None of the disorders in the group satisfies the criteria for either manic (F30.–) or depressive (F32.–) episodes, although emotional changes and individual affective symptoms may be prominent from time to time.

These disorders are also defined by the absence of organic causation, such as states of concussion, delirium, or dementia. Perplexity, preoccupation, and inattention to the immediate conversation are often present, but if they are so marked or persistent as to suggest delirium or dementia of organic cause, the diagnosis should be delayed until investigation or observation has clarified this point. Similarly, disorders in F23.– should not be diagnosed in the presence of obvious intoxication by drugs or alcohol. However, a recent minor increase in the consumption of, for instance, alcohol or marijuana, with no evidence of severe intoxication or disorientation, should not rule out the diagnosis of one of these acute psychotic disorders.

It is important to note that the 48–hour and the 2–week criteria are not put forward as the times of maximum severity and disturbance, but as times by which the psychotic symptoms have become obvious and disruptive of at least some aspects of daily life and work. The peak disturbance may be reached later in both instances; the symptoms and disturbance have only to be obvious by the stated times, in the sense that they will usually have brought the patient into contact with some form of helping or medical agency. Prodromal periods of anxiety, depression, social withdrawal, or mildly abnormal behaviour do not qualify for inclusion in these periods of time.

A fifth character may be used to indicate whether or nor the acute psychotic disorder is associated with acute stress:

F23.x0   Without associated acute stress
F23.x1   With associated acute stress

F23.0   *Acute polymorphic psychotic disorder without symptoms of schizophrenia*
An acute psychotic disorder in which hallucinations, delusions, and perceptual disturbances are obvious but markedly variable, changing from day to day or even from hour to hour. Emotional turmoil, with intense transient feelings of happiness and ecstasy or anxieties and irritability, is also frequently present. This polymorphic and unstable, changing clinical picture is characteristic, and even though individual affective or psychotic symptoms may at times be present, the criteria for manic episode (F30.–), depressive episode (F32.–), or schizophrenia (F20.–) are not fulfilled. This disorder is particularly likely to have an abrupt onset (within 48 hours) and a rapid resolution of symptoms; in a large proportion of cases there is no obvious precipitating stress.

If the symptoms persist for more than 3 months, the diagnosis should be changed. (Persistent delusional disorder (F22.–) or other nonorganic psychotic disorder (F28) is likely to be the most appropriate.)

Diagnostic guidelines

For a definite diagnosis:

(a) the onset must be acute (from a nonpsychotic state to a clearly psychotic state within 2 weeks or less);

(b) there must be several types of hallucination or delusion, changing in both type and intensity from day to day or within the same day;

(c) there should be a similarly varying emotional state; and

(d) in spite of the variety of symptoms, none should be present with sufficient consistency to fulfil the criteria for schizophrenia (F20.–) or for manic or depressive episode, (F30.– or F32.–).

Includes: *bouffée délirante* without symptoms of schizophrenia or unspecified
cycloid psychosis without symptoms of schizophrenia or unspecified

F23.1 *Acute polymorphic psychotic disorder with symptoms of schizophrenia*
An acute psychotic disorder that meets the descriptive criteria for acute polymorphic psychotic disorder (F23.0) but in which typically schizophrenic symptoms are also consistently present.

Diagnostic guidelines

For a definite diagnosis, criteria (a), (b), and (c) specified for acute polymorphic psychotic disorder (F23.0) must be fulfilled; in addition, symptoms that fulfil the criteria for schizophrenia (F20.–) must have been present for the majority of the time since the establishment of an obviously psychotic clinical picture.

If the schizophrenic symptoms persist for more than 1 month, the diagnosis should be changed to schizophrenia (F20.–).

Includes: *bouffée délirante* with symptoms of schizophrenia
cycloid psychosis with symptoms of schizophrenia

F23.2 *Acute schizophrenia-like psychotic disorder*
An acute psychotic disorder in which the psychotic symptoms are comparatively stable and fulfil the criteria for schizophrenia (F20.–) but have lasted for less than 1 month. Some degree of emotional variability or instability may be present, but not to the extent described in acute polymorphic psychotic disorder (F23.0).

Diagnostic guidelines
For a definite diagnosis:

(a) the onset of psychotic symptoms must be acute (2 weeks or less from a nonpsychotic to a clearly psychotic state);

(b) symptoms that fulfil the criteria for schizophrenia (F20.–) must have been present for the majority of the time since the establishment of an obviously psychotic clinical picture;

(c) the criteria for acute polymorphic psychotic disorder are not fulfilled.
If the schizophrenic symptoms last for more than 1 month, the diagnosis should be changed to schizophrenia (F20.–).

Includes: acute (undifferentiated) schizophrenia
brief schizophreniform disorder
brief schizophreniform psychosis
oneirophrenia
schizophrenic reaction

Excludes: organic delusional [schizophrenia-like] disorder (F06.2)
schizophreniform disorder NOS (F20.8)

F23.3   ***Other acute predominantly delusional psychotic disorders***
Acute psychotic disorders in which comparatively stable delusions or hallucinations are the main clinical features, but do not fulfil the criteria for schizophrenia (F20.–). Delusions of persecution or reference are common, and hallucinations are usually auditory (voices talking directly to the patient).

Diagnostic guidelines
For a definite diagnosis:

(a) the onset of psychotic symptoms must be acute (2 weeks or less from a nonpsychotic to a clearly psychotic state);

(b) delusions or hallucinations must have been present for the majority of the time since the establishment of an obviously psychotic state; and

(c) the criteria for neither schizophrenia (F20.–) nor acute polymorphic psychotic disorder (F23.0) are fulfilled.

If delusions persist for more than 3 months, the diagnosis should be changed to persistent delusional disorder (F22.–). If only hallucinations persist for more than 3 months, the diagnosis should be changed to other nonorganic psychotic disorder (F28).

Includes: paranoid reaction
     psychogenic paranoid psychosis

F23.8 *Other acute and transient psychotic disorders*

Any other acute psychotic disorders that are unclassifiable under any other category in F23 (such as acute psychotic states in which definite delusions or hallucinations occur but persist for only small proportions of the time) should be coded here. States of undifferentiated excitement should also be coded here if more detailed information about the patient's mental state is not available, provided that there is no evidence of an organic cause.

F23.9 *Acute and transient psychotic disorder, unspecified*

Includes: (brief) reactive psychosis NOS

F24 **Induced delusional disorder**

A delusional disorder shared by two or more people with close emotional links. Only one of the people suffers from a genuine psychotic disorder; the delusions are induced in the other(s) and usually disappear when the people are separated.

Includes: *folie à deux*
     induced paranoid or psychotic disorder

F25 **Schizoaffective disorders**

These are episodic disorders in which both affective and schizophrenic symptoms are prominent within the same episode of illness, preferably simultaneously, but at least within a few days of each other. Their relationship to typical mood [affective] disorders (F30–F39) and to schizophrenic disorders (F20–F24) is uncertain. They are given a separate category because they are too common to be ignored. Other conditions in which affective symptoms are superimposed upon or form part of a pre-existing schizophrenic illness, or in which they coexist or alternate with other types of persistent delusional disorders, are classified under the appropriate category in F20–F29. Mood-incongruent delusions or hallucinations in affective disorders (F30.2, F31.2, F31.5, F32.3, or F33.3) do not by themselves justify a diagnosis of schizoaffective disorder.

Patients who suffer from recurrent schizoaffective episodes, particularly those whose symptoms are of the manic rather than the depressive type, usually make a full recovery and only rarely develop a defect state.

Diagnostic guidelines

A diagnosis of schizoaffective disorder should be made only when *both* definite schizophrenic and definite affective symptoms are prominent *simultaneously*, or within a few days of each other, within the same episode of illness, and when, as a consequence of this, the episode of illness does not meet criteria for either schizophrenia or a depressive or manic episode. The term should not be applied to patients who exhibit schizophrenic symptoms and affective symptoms only in different episodes of illness. It is common, for example, for a schizophrenic patient to present with depressive symptoms in the aftermath of a psychotic episode (see post-schizophrenic depression (F20.4)). Some patients have recurrent schizoaffective episodes, which may be of the manic or depressive type or a mixture of the two. Others have one or two schizoaffective episodes interspersed between typical episodes of mania or depression. In the former case, schizoaffective disorder is the appropriate diagnosis. In the latter, the occurrence of an occasional schizoaffective episode does not invalidate a diagnosis of bipolar affective disorder or recurrent depressive disorder if the clinical picture is typical in other respects.

F25.0   Schizoaffective disorder, manic type

A disorder in which schizophrenic and manic symptoms are both prominent in the same episode of illness. The abnormality of mood usually takes the form of elation, accompanied by increased self-esteem and grandiose ideas, but sometimes excitement or irritability are more obvious and accompanied by aggressive behaviour and persecutory ideas. In both cases there is increased energy, overactivity, impaired concentration, and a loss of normal social inhibition. Delusions of reference, grandeur, or persecution may be present, but other more typically schizophrenic symptoms are required to establish the diagnosis. People may insist, for example, that their thoughts are being broadcast or interfered with, or that alien forces are trying to control them, or they may report hearing voices of varied kinds or express bizarre delusional ideas that are not merely grandiose or persecutory. Careful questioning is often required to establish that an individual really is experiencing these morbid phenomena, and not merely joking or talking in metaphors. Schizoaffective disorders, manic type, are usually florid psychoses with an acute onset; although behaviour is often grossly disturbed, full recovery generally occurs within a few weeks.

Diagnostic guidelines

There must be a prominent elevation of mood, or a less obvious elevation of mood combined with increased irritability or excitement. Within the same episode, at least one and preferably two typically schizophrenic symptoms (as specified for schizophrenia (F20.–), diagnostic guidelines (a)–(d)) should be clearly present.

This category should be used both for a single schizoaffective episode of the manic type and for a recurrent disorder in which the majority of episodes are schizoaffective, manic type.

Includes: schizoaffective psychosis, manic type
             schizophreniform psychosis, manic type

F25.1   Schizoaffective disorder, depressive type

A disorder in which schizophrenic and depressive symptoms are both prominent in the same episode of illness. Depression of mood is usually accompanied by several characteristic depressive symptoms or behavioural abnormalities such as retardation, insomnia, loss of energy, appetite or weight, reduction of normal interests, impairment of concentration, guilt, feelings of hopelessness, and suicidal thoughts. At the same time, or within the same episode, other more typically schizophrenic symptoms are present; patients may insist, for example, that their thoughts are being broadcast or interfered with, or that alien forces are trying to control them. They may be convinced that they are being spied upon or plotted against and this is not justified by their own behaviour. Voices may be heard that are not merely disparaging or condemnatory but that talk of killing the patient or discuss this behaviour between themselves. Schizoaffective episodes of the depressive type are usually less florid and alarming than schizoaffective episodes of the manic type, but they tend to last longer and the prognosis is less favourable. Although the majority of patients recover completely, some eventually develop a schizophrenic defect.

Diagnostic guidelines

There must be prominent depression, accompanied by at least two characteristic depressive symptoms or associated behavioural abnormalities as listed for depressive episode (F32.–); within the same episode, at least one and preferably two typically schizophrenic symptoms (as specified for schizophrenia (F20.–), diagnostic guidelines (a)–(d)) should be clearly present.

This category should be used both for a single schizoaffective episode, depressive type, and for a recurrent disorder in which the majority of episodes are schizoaffective, depressive type.

Includes: schizoaffective psychosis, depressive type
          schizophreniform psychosis, depressive type

F25.2 *Schizoaffective disorder, mixed type*
Disorders in which symptoms of schizophrenia (F20.–) coexist with those of a mixed bipolar affective disorder (F31.6) should be coded here.

Includes: cyclic schizophrenia
          mixed schizophrenic and affective psychosis

F25.8 *Other schizoaffective disorders*

F25.9 *Schizoaffective disorder, unspecified*
Includes: schizoaffective psychosis NOS

F28   Other nonorganic psychotic disorders

Psychotic disorders that do not meet the criteria for schizophrenia (F20.–) or for psychotic types of mood [affective] disorders (F30–F39), and psychotic disorders that do not meet the symptomatic criteria for persistent delusional disorder (F22.–) should be coded here.
Includes: chronic hallucinatory psychosis NOS

F29   Unspecified nonorganic psychosis

This category should also be used for psychosis of unknown etiology.
Includes: psychosis NOS
Excludes: mental disorder NOS (F99)
          organic or symptomatic psychosis NOS (F09)

F30–F39   **Mood [affective] disorders**

F30   Manic Episode

    F30.0   Hypomania

    F30.1   Mania without psychotic symptoms

    F30.2   Mania with psychotic symptoms

    F30.8   Other manic episodes

    F30.9   Manic episode, unspecified

F31   Bipolar affective disorder

    F31.0   Bipolar affective disorder, current episode hypomanic

    F31.1   Bipolar affective disorder, current episode manic without psychotic symptoms

    F31.2   Bipolar affective disorder, current episode manic with psychotic symptoms

    F31.3   Bipolar affective disorder, current episode mild or moderate depression

        .30   Without somatic syndrome

        .31   With somatic syndrome

    F31.4   Bipolar affective disorder, current episode severe depression without psychotic symptoms

    F31.5   Bipolar affective disorder, current episode severe depression with psychotic symptoms

    F31.6   Bipolar affective disorder, current episode mixed

    F31.7   Bipolar affective disorder, currently in remission

    F31.8   Other bipolar affective disorders

    F31.9   Bipolar affective disorder, unspecified

F32   Depressive episode

    F32.0   Mild depressive episode

        .00   Without somatic syndrome

        .01   With somatic syndrome

    F32.1   Moderate depressive episode

        .10   Without somatic syndrome

        .11   With somatic syndrome

    F32.2   Severe depressive episode without psychotic symptoms

    F32.3   Severe depressive episode with psychotic symptoms

    F32.8   Other depressive episodes

    F32.9   Depressive episode, unspecified

F33   Recurrent depressive disorder

    F33.0   Recurrent depressive disorder, current episode mild

        .00   Without somatic syndrome

        .01   With somatic syndrome

F33.1   Recurrent depressive disorder, current episode moderate
.10   Without somatic syndrome
.11   With somatic syndrome
F33.2   Recurrent depressive disorder, current episode severe without psychotic symptoms
F33.3   Recurrent depressive disorder, current episode severe with psychotic symptoms
F33.4   Recurrent depressive disorder, currently in remission
F33.8   Other recurrent depressive disorders
F33.9   Recurrent depressive disorder, unspecified

F34   Persistent mood [affective] disorders
F34.0   Cyclothymia
F34.1   Dysthymia
F34.8   Other persistent mood [affective] disorders
F34.9   Persistent mood [affective] disorder, unspecified

F38   Other mood [affective] disorders
F38.0   Other single mood [affective] disorders
.00   Mixed affective episode
F38.1   Other recurrent mood [affective] disorders
.10   Recurrent brief depressive disorder
F38.8   Other specified mood [affective] disorders

F39   Unspecified mood [affective] disorder

Introduction

The relationship between etiology, symptoms, underlying biochemical processes, response to treatment, and outcome of mood [affective] disorders is not yet sufficiently well understood to allow their classification in a way that is likely to meet with universal approval. Nevertheless, a classification must be attempted, and that presented here is put forward in the hope that it will at least be acceptable, since it is the result of widespread consultation.

In these disorders, the fundamental disturbance is a change in mood or affect, usually to depression (with or without associated anxiety) or to elation. This mood change is normally accompanied by a change in the overall level of activity, and most other symptoms are either secondary to, or easily understood in the context of, such changes. Most of these disorders tend to be recurrent, and the onset of individual episodes is often related to stressful events or situations. This block deals with mood

One

disorders in all age groups; those arising in childhood and adolescence should therefore be coded here.

The main criteria by which the affective disorders have been classified have been chosen for practical reasons, in that they allow common clinical disorders to be identified easily. Single episodes have been distinguished from bipolar and other multiple episode disorders because substantial proportions of patients have only one episode of illness, and severity is given prominence because of implications for treatment and for provision of different levels of service. It is acknowledged that the symptoms referred to here as 'somatic' could also have been called 'melancholic', 'vital', 'biological', or 'endogenomorphic', and that the scientific status of this syndrome is in any case somewhat questionable. It is to be hoped that the result of its inclusion here will be widespread critical appraisal of the usefulness of its separate identification. The classification is arranged so that this somatic syndrome can be recorded by those who so wish, but can also be ignored without loss of any other information.

Distinguishing between different grades of severity remains a problem; the three grades of mild, moderate, and severe have been specified here because many clinicians wish to have them available.

The terms 'mania' and 'severe depression' are used in this classification to denote the opposite ends of the affective spectrum; 'hypomania' is used to denote an intermediate state without delusions, hallucinations, or complete disruption of normal activities, which is often (but not exclusively) seen as patients develop or recover from mania.

F30   Manic episode

Three degrees of severity are specified here, sharing the common underlying characteristics of elevated mood, and an increase in the quantity and speed of physical and mental activity. All the subdivisions of this category should be used only for a single manic episode. If previous or subsequent affective episodes (depressive, manic, or hypomanic), the disorder should be coded under bipolar affective disorder (F31.–).

Includes: bipolar disorder, single manic episode

F30.0   *Hypomania*

Hypomania is a lesser degree of mania (F30.1), in which abnormalities of mood and behaviour are too persistent and marked to be included under cyclothymia (F34.0) but are not accompanied by hallucinations or delusions. There is a persistent mild elevation of mood (for at least several days on end), increased energy and activity, and usually marked feelings of well-being and both physical and mental efficiency. Increased sociability, talkativeness, overfamiliarity, increased sexual energy, and a decreased need for sleep are often present but not to the extent that they lead to severe disruption of work or result in social rejection. Irritability, conceit, and boorish behaviour may take the place of the more usual euphoric sociability.

Concentration and attention may be impaired, thus diminishing the ability to settle down to work or to relaxation and leisure, but this may not prevent the appearance of interests in quite new ventures and activities, or mild over-spending.

Diagnostic guidelines
Several of the features mentioned above, consistent with elevated or changed mood and increased activity, should be present for at least several days on end, to a degree and with a persistence greater than described for cyclothymia (F34.0). Considerable interference with work or social activity is consistent with a diagnosis of hypomania, but if disruption of these is severe or complete, mania (F30.1 or F30.2) should be diagnosed.

Differential diagnosis
Hypomania covers the range of disorders of mood and level of activities between cyclothymia (F34.0) and mania (F30.1 and F30.2). The increased activity and restlessness (and often weight loss) must be distinguished from the same symptoms occurring in hyperthyroidism and anorexia nervosa; early states of 'agitated depression' may bear a superficial resemblance to hypomania of the irritable variety (although this is more likely to be seen in late middle age). Patients with severe obsessional symptoms may be active part of the night completing their domestic cleaning rituals, but their affect will usually be the opposite of that described here.

When a short period of hypomania occurs as a prelude to or aftermath of mania (F30.1 and F30.2), it is usually not worth specifying the hypomania separately.

F30.1   Mania without psychotic symptoms
Mood is elevated out of keeping with the individual's circumstances and may vary from carefree joviality to almost uncontrollable excitement. Elation is accompanied by increased energy, resulting in overactivity,

pressure of speech, and a decreased need for sleep. Normal social inhibitions are lost, attention cannot be sustained, and there is often marked distractibility. Self-esteem is inflated, and grandiose or over-optimistic ideas are freely expressed.

Perceptual disorders may occur, such as the appreciation of colours as especially vivid (and usually beautiful), a preoccupation with fine details of surfaces or textures, and subjective hyperacusis. The individual may embark on extravagant and impractical schemes, spend money recklessly, or become aggressive, amorous, or facetious in inappropriate circumstances. In some manic episodes the mood is irritable and suspicious rather than elated. The first attack occurs most commonly between the ages of 15 and 30 years, but may occur at any age from late childhood onwards.

Diagnostic guidelines
The episode should last for at least 1 week and should be severe enough to disrupt ordinary work and social activities more or less completely. The mood change should be accompanied by increased energy and several of the symptoms referred to above (particularly pressure of speech, decreased need for sleep, grandiosity, and excessive optimism).

F30.2   *Mania with psychotic symptoms*
The clinical picture is that of a more severe form of mania as described in F30.1. Inflated self-esteem and grandiose ideas may develop into delusions, and irritability and suspiciousness into delusions of persecution. In severe cases, grandiose or religious delusions of identity or role may be prominent, and flight of ideas and pressure of speech may result in the individual becoming incomprehensible. Severe and sustained physical activity and excitement may result in aggression or violence, and neglect of eating, drinking, and personal hygiene may result in dangerous states of dehydration and self-neglect. If required, delusions or hallucinations can be specified as congruent or incongruent with the mood. 'Incongruent' should be taken as including affectively neutral delusions and hallucinations; for example, delusions of reference with no guilty or accusatory content, or voices speaking to the individual about events that have no special emotional significance.

Differential diagnosis
One of the commonest problems is differentiation of this disorder from schizophrenia, particularly if the stages of development through hypoma-

nia have been missed and the patient is seen only at the height of the illness when widespread delusions, incomprehensible speech, and violent excitement may obscure the basic disturbance of affect. Patients with mania that is responding to neuroleptic medication may present a similar diagnostic problem at the stage when they have returned to normal levels of physical and mental activity but still have delusions or hallucinations. Occasional hallucinations or delusions as specified for schizophrenia (F20.–) may also be classed as mood-incongruent, but if these symptoms are prominent and persistent, the diagnosis of schizoaffective disorder (F25.–) is more likely to be appropriate.

Includes: manic stupor

F30.8   *Other manic episodes*

F30.9   *Manic episode, unspecified*
Includes: mania NOS

F31   Bipolar affective disorder

This disorder is characterized by repeated (i.e. at least two) episodes in which the patient's mood and activity levels are significantly disturbed, this disturbance consisting on some occasions of an elevation of mood and increased energy and activity (mania or hypomania), and on others of a lowering of mood and decreased energy and activity (depression). Characteristically, recovery is usually complete between episodes, and the incidence in the two sexes is more nearly equal than in other mood disorders. As patients who suffer only from repeated episodes of mania are comparatively rare, and resemble (in their family history, premorbid personality, age of onset, and long-term prognosis) those who also have at least occasional episodes of depression, such patients are classified as bipolar (F31.8).

Manic episodes usually begin abruptly and last for between 2 weeks and 4–5 months (median duration about 4 months). Depressions tend to last longer (median length about 6 months), though rarely for more than a year. Episodes of both kinds often follow stressful life events or other mental trauma, but the presence of such stress is not essential for the diagnosis. The first episode may occur at any age from childhood onwards. The frequency of episodes and the pattern of remissions and relapses are both very variable, though remissions tend to get shorter as time goes on and depressions to become commoner and longer lasting after middle age.

Although the original concept of 'manic-depressive psychosis' also included patients who suffered only from depression, the term 'manic-depressive disorder or psychosis' is now used mainly as a synonym for bipolar disorder.

Includes: manic-depressive illness, psychosis or reaction
Excludes: bipolar disorder, single manic episode (F30.–)
         cyclothymia (F34.0)

F31.0 *Bipolar affective disorder, current episode hypomanic*

Diagnostic guidelines
For a definite diagnosis:

(a) the current episode must fulfil the criteria for hypomania (F30.0); and
(b) there must have been at least one other affective episode (hypomanic, manic, depressive, or mixed) in the past.

F31.1 *Bipolar affective disorder, current episode manic without psychotic symptoms*

Diagnostic guidelines
For a definite diagnosis:

(a) the current episode must fulfil the criteria for mania without psychotic symptoms (F30.1); and
(b) there must have been at least one other affective episode (hypomanic, manic, depressive, or mixed) in the past.

F31.2 *Bipolar affective disorder, current episode manic with psychotic symptoms*

Diagnostic guidelines
For a definite diagnosis:

(a) the current episode must fulfil the criteria for mania with psychotic symptoms (F30.2); and
(b) there must have been at least one other affective episode (hypomanic, manic, depressive, or mixed) in the past.

If required, delusions or hallucinations may be specified as congruent or incongruent with mood (see F30.2).

F31.3   *Bipolar affective disorder, current episode mild or moderate depression*

Diagnostic guidelines
For a definite diagnosis:

(a)   the current episode must fulfil the criteria for a depressive episode of either mild (F32.0) or moderate (F32.1) severity; and

(b)   there must have been at least one hypomanic, manic, or mixed affective episode in the past.

A fifth character may be used to specify the presence or absence of the somatic syndrome in the current episode of depression:

F31.30 Without somatic syndrome
F31.31 With somatic syndrome

F31.4   *Bipolar affective disorder, current episode severe depression without psychotic symptoms*

Diagnostic guidelines
For a definite diagnosis:

(a)   the current episode must fulfil the criteria for a severe depressive episode without psychotic symptoms (F32.2); and

(b)   there must have been at least one hypomanic, manic, or mixed affective episode in the past.

F31.5   *Bipolar affective disorder, current episode severe depression with psychotic symptoms*

Diagnostic guidelines
For a definite diagnosis:

(a)   the current episode must fulfil the criteria for a severe depressive episode with psychotic symptoms (F32.3); and

(b)   there must have been at least one hypomanic, manic, or mixed affective episode in the past.

If required, delusions or hallucinations may be specified as congruent or incongruent with mood (see F30.2).

F31.6   Bipolar affective disorder, current episode mixed

The patient has had at least one manic, hypomanic, or mixed affective episode in the past and currently exhibits either a mixture or a rapid alternation of manic, hypomanic, and depressive symptoms.

Diagnostic guidelines

Although the most typical form of bipolar disorder consists of alternating manic and depressive episodes separated by periods of normal mood, it is not uncommon for depressive mood to be accompanied for days or weeks on end by overactivity and pressure of speech, or for a manic mood and grandiosity to be accompanied by agitation and loss of energy and libido. Depressive symptoms and symptoms of hypomania or mania may also alternate rapidly, from day to day or even from hour to hour. A diagnosis of mixed bipolar affective disorder should be made only if the two sets of symptoms are both prominent for the greater part of the current episode of illness, and if that episode has lasted for at least 2 weeks.

Excludes: single mixed affective episode (F38.0)

F31.7   Bipolar affective disorder, currently in remission

The patient has had at least one manic, hypomanic, or mixed affective episode in the past and in addition at least one other affective episode of hypomanic, manic, depressive, or mixed type, but is not currently suffering from any significant mood disturbance, and has not done so for several months. The patient may, however, be receiving treatment to reduce the risk of future episodes.

F31.8   Other bipolar affective disorders

Includes: bipolar II disorder
              recurrent manic episodes

F31.9   Bipolar affective disorder, unspecified

F32   Depressive episode

In typical depressive episodes of all three varieties described below (mild (F32.0), moderate (F32.1), and severe (F32.2 and F32.3)), the individual usually suffers from depressed mood, loss of interest and enjoyment, and reduced energy leading to increased fatiguability and diminished activity. Marked tiredness after only slight effort is common. Other common symptoms are:

(a) reduced concentration and attention;
(b) reduced self-esteem and self-confidence;
(c) ideas of guilt and unworthiness (even in a mild type of episode);
(d) bleak and pessimistic views of the future;
(e) ideas or acts of self-harm or suicide;
(f) disturbed sleep;
(g) diminished appetite.

The lowered mood varies little from day to day, and is often unresponsive to circumstances, yet may show a characteristic diurnal variation as the day goes on. As with manic episodes, the clinical presentation shows marked individual variations, and atypical presentations are particularly common in adolescence. In some cases, anxiety, distress, and motor agitation may be more prominent at times than the depression, and the mood change may also be masked by added features such as irritability, excessive consumption of alcohol, histrionic behaviour, and exacerbation of pre-existing phobic or obsessional symptoms, or by hypochondriacal preoccupations. For depressive episodes of all three grades of severity, a duration of at least 2 weeks is usually required for diagnosis, but shorter periods may be reasonable if symptoms are unusually severe and of rapid onset.

Some of the above symptoms may be marked and develop characteristic features that are widely regarded as having special clinical significance. The most typical examples of these 'somatic' symptoms are: loss of interest or pleasure in activities that are normally enjoyable; lack of emotional reactivity to normally pleasurable surroundings and events; waking in the morning 2 hours or more before the usual time; depression worse in the morning; objective evidence of definite psychomotor retardation or agitation (remarked on or reported by other people); marked loss of appetite; weight loss (often defined as 5% or more of body weight in the past month); marked loss of libido. Usually, this somatic syndrome is not regarded as present unless about four of these symptoms are definitely present.

The categories of mild (F32.0), moderate (F32.1) and severe (F32.2 and F32.3) depressive episodes described in more detail below should be used only for a single (first) depressive episode. Further depressive episodes should be classified under one of the subdivisions of recurrent depressive disorder (F33.–).

These grades of severity are specified to cover a wide range of clinical states that are encountered in different types of psychiatric practice.

Individuals with mild depressive episodes are common in primary care and general medical settings, whereas psychiatric inpatient units deal largely with patients suffering from the severe grades.

Acts of self-harm associated with mood [affective] disorders, most commonly self-poisoning by prescribed medication, should be recorded by means of an additional code from Chapter XX of ICD-10 (X60–X84). These codes do not involve differentiation between attempted suicide and 'parasuicide', since both are included in the general category of self-harm.

Differentiation between mild, moderate, and severe depressive episodes rests upon a complicated clinical judgement that involves the number, type, and severity of symptoms present. The extent of ordinary social and work activities is often a useful general guide to the likely degree of severity of the episode, but individual, social, and cultural influences that disrupt a smooth relationship between severity of symptoms and social performance are sufficiently common and powerful to make it unwise to include social performance amongst the essential criteria of severity.

The presence of dementia (F00–F03) or mental retardation (F70–F79) does not rule out the diagnosis of a treatable depressive episode, but communication difficulties are likely to make it necessary to rely more than usual for the diagnosis upon objectively observed somatic symptoms, such as psychomotor retardation, loss of appetite and weight, and sleep disturbance.

Includes: single episodes of depressive reaction, major depression (without psychotic symptoms), psychogenic depression or reactive depression (F32.0, F32.1 or F32.2)

F32.0   *Mild depressive episode*

Diagnostic guidelines
Depressed mood, loss of interest and enjoyment, and increased fatiguability are usually regarded as the most typical symptoms of depression, and at least two of these, plus at least two of the other symptoms described should usually be present for a definite diagnosis. None of the symptoms should be present to an intense degree. Minimum duration of the whole episode is about 2 weeks.

An individual with a mild depressive episode is usually distressed by the symptoms and has some difficulty in continuing with ordinary work and social activities, but will probably not cease to function completely.

A fifth character may be used to specify the presence of a somatic syndrome:

F32.00 Without somatic syndrome
The criteria for mild depressive episode are fulfilled, and there are few or none of the somatic symptoms present.

F32.01 With somatic syndrome
The criteria for mild depressive episode are fulfilled, and four or more of the somatic symptoms are also present. (If only two or three somatic symptoms are present but they are unusually severe, use of this category may be justified.)

F32.1   *Moderate depressive episode*

Diagnostic guidelines
At least two of the three most typical symptoms noted for mild depressive episode (F32.0) should be present, plus at least three (and preferably four) of the other symptoms. Several symptoms are likely to be present to a marked degree, but this is not essential if a particularly wide variety of symptoms is present overall. Minimum duration of the whole episode is about 2 weeks.

An individual with a moderately severe depressive episode will usually have considerable difficulty in continuing with social, work or domestic activities.

A fifth character may be used to specify the occurrence of the somatic syndrome:

F32.10 Without somatic syndrome
The criteria for moderate depressive episode are fulfilled, and few if any of the somatic symptoms are present.

F32.11 With somatic syndrome
The criteria for moderate depressive episode are fulfilled, and four or more or the somatic symptoms are present. (If only two or three somatic symptoms are present but they are unusually severe, use of this category may be justified.)

F32.2   *Severe depressive episode without psychotic symptoms*
In a severe depressive episode, the sufferer usually shows considerable distress or agitation, unless retardation is a marked feature. Loss of self-

One

esteem or feelings of uselessness or guilt are likely to be prominent, and suicide is a distinct danger in particularly severe cases. It is presumed here that the somatic syndrome will almost always be present in a severe depressive episode.

Diagnostic guidelines

All three of the typical symptoms noted for mild and moderate depressive episodes (F32.0, F32.1) should be present, plus at least four other symptoms, some of which should be of severe intensity. However, if important symptoms such as agitation or retardation are marked, the patient may be unwilling or unable to describe many symptoms in detail. An overall grading of severe episode may still be justified in such instances. The depressive episode should usually last at least 2 weeks, but if the symptoms are particularly severe and of very rapid onset, it may be justified to make this diagnosis after less than 2 weeks.

During a severe depressive episode it is very unlikely that the sufferer will be able to continue with social, work, or domestic activities, except to a very limited extent.

This category should be used only for single episodes of severe depression without psychotic symptoms; for further episodes, a subcategory of recurrent depressive disorder (F33.–) should be used.

Includes: single episodes of agitated depression
melancholia or vital depression without psychotic symptoms

F32.3   *Severe depressive episode with psychotic symptoms*

Diagnostic guidelines

A severe depressive episode which meets the criteria given for F32.2 above and in which delusions, hallucinations, or depressive stupor are present. The delusions usually involve ideas of sin, poverty, or imminent disasters, responsibility for which may be assumed by the patient. Auditory or olfactory hallucinations are usually of defamatory or accusatory voices or of rotting filth or decomposing flesh. Severe psychomotor retardation may progress to stupor. If required, delusions or hallucinations may be specified as mood-congruent or mood-incongruent (see F30.2).

Differential diagnosis

Depressive stupor must be differentiated from catatonic schizophrenia (F20.2), from dissociative stupor (F44.2), and from organic forms of stupor. This category should be used only for single episodes of severe depression with psychotic symptoms; for further episodes a subcategory of recurrent depressive disorder (F33.–) should be used.

Includes: single episodes of major depression with psychotic symptoms, psychotic depression, psychogenic depressive psychosis, reactive depressive psychosis

F32.8   *Other depressive episodes*

Episodes should be included here which do not fit the descriptions given for depressive episodes described in F32.0–F32.3, but for which the overall diagnostic impression indicates that they are depressive in nature. Examples include fluctuating mixtures of depressive symptoms (particularly the somatic variety) with non-diagnostic symptoms such as tension, worry, and distress, and mixtures of somatic depressive symptoms with persistent pain or fatigue not due to organic causes (as sometimes seen in general hospital services).

Includes: atypical depression
single episodes of 'masked' depression NOS

F32.9   *Depressive episode, unspecified*

Includes: depression NOS
depressive disorder NOS

F33   Recurrent depressive disorder

A disorder characterized by repeated episodes of depression as described in depressive episode (32.-), without any history of independent episodes of mood elevation and increased energy (mania). There may, however, be brief episodes of mild mood elevation and overactivity (hypomania) immediately after a depressive episode, sometimes precipitated by antidepressant treatment. The more severe forms of recurrent depressive disorder (33.2 and 33.3) have much in common with earlier concepts such as manic-depressive depression, melancholia, vital depression and endogenous depression. The first episode may occur at any age from childhood to old age, the onset may be either acute or insidious, and the duration varies from a few weeks to many months. The risk that a patient with recurrent depressive disorder will have an episode of mania never disappears completely, however many depressive episodes have been experienced. If such an episode does occur, the diagnosis should be changed to bipolar affective disorder (31.-).

One

Includes: recurrent episodes of:
depressive reaction
psychogenic depression
reactive depression
seasonal depressive disorder
Excludes: recurrent brief depressive episodes (38.1)

F33.0 ***Recurrent depressive disorder, current episode mild***
A disorder characterized by repeated episodes of depression, the current episode being mild, as in 32.0, and without any history of mania.

F33.1 ***Recurrent depressive disorder, current episode moderate***
A disorder characterized by repeated episodes of depression, the current episode being of moderate severity, as in 32.1, and without any history of mania.

F33.2 ***Recurrent depressive disorder, current episode severe without psychotic symptoms***
A disorder characterized by repeated episodes of depression, the current episode being severe without psychotic symptoms, as in 32.2, and without any history of mania.

Endogenous depression without psychotic symptoms
Major depression, recurrent without psychotic symptoms
Manic-depressive psychosis, depressed type without psychotic symptoms
Vital depression, recurrent without psychotic symptoms

F33.3 ***Recurrent depressive disorder, current episode severe with psychotic symptoms***
A disorder characterized by repeated episodes of depression, the current episode being severe with psychotic symptoms, as in 32.3, and without any previous episodes of mania.

Includes: endogenous depression with psychotic symptoms
manic-depressive psychosis, depressed type with psychotic symptoms
recurrent severe episodes of:
major depression with psychotic symptoms
psychogenic depressive psychosis
psychotic depression
reactive depressive psychosis

F33.4   Recurrent depressive disorder, currently in remission
The patient has had two or more depressive episodes as described in 33.0-33.3, in the past, but has been free from depressive symptoms for several months.

F33.8   Other recurrent depressive disorders

F33.9   Recurrent depressive disorder, unspecified
Monopolar depression NOS

F34   Persistent mood [affective] disorders
Persistent and usually fluctuating disorders of mood in which the majority of the individual episodes are not sufficiently severe to warrant being described as hypomanic or mild depressive episodes. Because they last for years on end, and sometimes for the greater part of the patient's adult life, they involve considerable distress and disability. In some instances, recurrent or single manic or depressive episodes may become superimposed on a persistent affective disorder. Therefore, the latter diagnosis and the diagnosis of any one of the affective disorders 30-33 are not mutually exclusive.

F34.0   Cyclothymia
A persistent instability of mood involving numerous periods of depression and mild elation (hypomania), none of which is sufficiently severe or prolonged to justify a diagnosis of bipolar affective disorder (31.-) or recurrent depressive disorder (33.-). This disorder is frequently found in the relatives of patients with bipolar affective disorder. Some patients with cyclothymia eventually develop bipolar affective disorder.

Affective personality disorder
Cycloid personality
Cyclothymic personality

F34.1   Dysthymia
A chronic depression of mood, lasting at least several years, which is not sufficiently severe, or in which individual episodes are not sufficiently prolonged, to justify a diagnosis of severe, moderate or mild recurrent depressive disorder (33.-).

Depressive:

> neurosis
>
> personality disorder

Neurotic depression

Persistent anxiety depression

Excludes: anxiety depression (mild or not persistent) (41.2)

F34.8   *Other persistent mood [affective] disorders*

F34.9   *Persistent mood [affective] disorder, unspecified*

F38   Other mood [affective] disorders

F38.0   *Other single mood [affective] disorders*

F38.00 Mixed affective episode
An affective episode lasting for at least 2 weeks, characterized by either a mixture or a rapid alternation (usually within a few hours) of hypomanic, manic, and depressive symptoms.

F38.1   *Other recurrent mood [affective] disorders*

F38.10 Recurrent brief depressive disorder
Recurrent brief depressive episodes, occurring about once a month over the past year. The individual depressive episodes all last less than 2 weeks (typically 2–3 days, with complete recovery) but fulfil the symptomatic criteria for mild, moderate, or severe depressive episode (F32.0, F32.1, F32.2).

Differential diagnosis
In contrast to those with dysthymia (F34.1), patients are not depressed for the majority of the time. If the depressive episodes occur only in relation to the menstrual cycle, F38.8 should be used with a second code for the underlying cause (N94.8, other specified conditions associated with female genital organs and menstrual cycle).

F38.8   *Other specified mood [affective] disorders*
This is a residual category for affective disorders that do not meet the criteria for any other categories F30–F38.1 above.

F39   Unspecified mood [affective] disorder

To be used only as a last resort, when no other term can be used.

Includes: affective psychosis NOS
Excludes: mental disorder NOS (F99)

F40–F48   **Neurotic, stress-related and somatoform disorders**

F40   Phobic anxiety disorders
  F40.0 Agoraphobia
   .00 Without panic disorder
   .01 With panic disorder
  F40.1 Social phobias
  F40.2 Specific (isolated) phobias
  F40.8 Other phobic anxiety disorders
  F40.9 Phobic anxiety disorder, unspecified

F41   Other anxiety disorders
  F41.0 Panic disorder [episodic paroxysmal anxiety]
  F41.1 Generalized anxiety disorder
  F41.2 Mixed anxiety and depressive disorder
  F41.3 Other mixed anxiety disorders
  F41.8 Other specified anxiety disorders
  F41.9 Anxiety disorder, unspecified

F42   Obsessive-compulsive disorder
  F42.0 Predominantly obsessional thoughts or ruminations
  F42.1 Predominantly compulsive acts [obsessional rituals]
  F42.2 Mixed obsessional thoughts and acts
  F42.8 Other obsessive-compulsive disorders
  F42.9 Obsessive-compulsive disorder, unspecified

F43   Reaction to severe stress, and adjustment disorders
  F43.0 Acute stress reaction
  F43.1 Post-traumatic stress disorder
  F43.2 Adjustment disorders
   .20 Brief depressive reaction
   .21 Prolonged depressive reaction
   .22 Mixed anxiety and depressive reaction
   .23 With predominant disturbance of other emotions
   .24 With predominant disturbance of conduct
   .25 With mixed disturbance of emotions and conduct
   .28 With other specified predominant symptoms
  F43.8 Other reactions to severe stress
  F43.9 Reaction to severe stress, unspecified

F44   Dissociative [conversion] disorders
  F44.0 Dissociative amnesia
  F44.1 Dissociative fugue

F44.2   Dissociative stupor
F44.3   Trance and possession disorders
F44.4   Dissociative motor disorders
F44.5   Dissociative convulsions
F44.6   Dissociative anæsthesia and sensory loss
F44.7   Mixed dissociative [conversion] disorders
F44.8   Other dissociative [conversion] disorders
  .80   Ganser's syndrome
  .81   Multiple personality disorder
  .82   Transient dissociative [conversion] disorders occurring in childhood and adolescence
  .88   Other specified dissociative [conversion] disorders
F44.9   Dissociative [conversion] disorder, unspecified

F45   Somatoform disorders
F45.0   Somatization disorder
F45.1   Undifferentiated somatoform disorder
F45.2   Hypochondriacal disorder
F45.3   Somatoform autonomic dysfunction
  .30   Heart and cardiovascular system
  .31   Upper gastrointestinal tract
  .32   Lower gastrointestinal tract
  .33   Respiratory system
  .34   Genitourinary system
  .38   Other organ or system
F45.4   Persistent somatoform pain disorder
F45.8   Other somatoform disorders
F45.9   Somatoform disorder, unspecified

F48   Other neurotic disorders
F48.0   Neurasthenia
F48.1   Depersonalization-derealization syndrome
F48.8   Other specified neurotic disorders
F48.9   Neurotic disorder, unspecified

Introduction

Neurotic, stress-related, and somatoform disorders have been brought together in one large overall group because of their historical association with the concept of neurosis and the association of a substantial (though uncertain) proportion of these disorders with psychological causation.

One

As noted in the general introduction to the *ICD-10 Classification of Mental and Behavioural Disorders: Clinical Descriptions and Diagnostic Guidelines*, the concept of neurosis has not been retained as a major organizing principle, but care has been taken to allow the easy identification of disorders that some users still might wish to regard as neurotic in their own usage of the term.

Mixtures of symptoms are common (coexistent depression and anxiety being by far the most frequent), particularly in the less severe varieties of these disorders often seen in primary care. Although efforts should be made to decide which is the predominant syndrome, a category is provided for those cases of mixed depression and anxiety in which it would be artificial to force a decision (F41.2).

F40   Phobic anxiety disorders

In this group of disorders, anxiety is evoked only, or predominantly, by certain well-defined situations or objects (external to the individual) that are not currently dangerous. As a result, these situations or objects are characteristically avoided or endured with dread. Phobic anxiety is indistinguishable subjectively, physiologically, and behaviourally from other types of anxiety and may vary in severity from mild unease to terror. The individual's concern may focus on individual symptoms such as palpitations or feeling faint and is often associated with secondary fears of dying, losing control, or going mad. The anxiety is not relieved by the knowledge that other people do not regard the situation in question as dangerous or threatening. Mere contemplation of entry to the phobic situation usually generates anticipatory anxiety.

The adoption of the criterion that the phobic object or situation is external to the subject implies that many of the fears relating to the presence of disease (nosophobia) and disfigurement (dysmorphobia) are now classified under F45.2 (hypochondriacal disorder). However, if the fear of disease arises predominantly and repeatedly from possible exposure to infection or contamination, or is simply a fear of medical procedures (injections, operations, etc.) or medical establishments (dentists' surgeries, hospitals, etc.), a category from F40.– will be appropriate (usually F40.2, specific phobia).

Phobic anxiety often coexists with depression. Pre-existing phobic anxiety almost invariably gets worse during an intercurrent depressive episode. Some depressive episodes are accompanied by temporary phobic anxiety and a depressive mood often accompanies some phobias, particularly agoraphobia. Whether two diagnoses, phobic anxiety and depressive episode, are needed or only one is determined by whether one disorder developed clearly before the other and by whether one is clearly predominant at the time of diagnosis. If the criteria for depressive disorder were met before the phobic symptoms first appeared, the former should be given diagnostic precedence (see note in Introduction, pages 6 and 7).

Most phobic disorders other than social phobias are more common in women than in men.

In this classification, a panic attack (F41.0) occurring in an established phobic situation is regarded as an expression of the severity of the phobia, which should be given diagnostic precedence. Panic disorder as a main diagnosis should be diagnosed only in the absence of any of the phobias listed in F40.–.

F40.0   Agoraphobia

The term 'agoraphobia' is used here with a wider meaning than it had when originally introduced and as it is still used in some countries. It is now taken to include fears not only of open spaces but also of related aspects such as the presence of crowds and the difficulty of immediate easy escape to a safe place (usually home). The term therefore refers to an interrelated and often overlapping cluster of phobias embracing fears of leaving home: fear of entering shops, crowds, and public places, or of travelling alone in trains, buses, or planes. Although the severity of the anxiety and the extent of avoidance behaviour are variable, this is the most incapacitating of the phobic disorders and some sufferers become completely housebound; many are terrified by the thought of collapsing and being left helpless in public. The lack of an immediately available exit is one of the key features of many of these agoraphobic situations. Most sufferers are women and the onset is usually early in adult life. Depressive and obsessional symptoms and social phobias may also be present but do not dominate the clinical picture. In the absence of effective treatment, agoraphobia often becomes chronic, though usually fluctuating.

Diagnostic guidelines

All of the following criteria should be fulfilled for a definite diagnosis:

(a)   the psychological or autonomic symptoms must be primarily manifestations of anxiety and not secondary to other symptoms, such as delusions or obsessional thoughts;

(b)   the anxiety must be restricted to (or occur mainly in) at least two of the following situations: crowds, public places, travelling away from home, and travelling alone; and

(c)   avoidance of the phobic situation must be, or have been, a prominent feature.

Differential diagnosis

It must be remembered that some agoraphobics experience little anxiety because they are consistently able to avoid their phobic situations. The presence of other symptoms such as depression, depersonalization, obsessional symptoms, and social phobias does not invalidate the diagnosis, provided that these symptoms do not dominate the clinical picture. However, if the patient was already significantly depressed when the phobic symptoms first appeared, depressive episode may be a more appropriate main diagnosis; this is more common in late-onset cases.

The presence or absence of panic disorder (F41.0) in the agoraphobic situation on a majority of occasions may be recorded by means of a fifth character:

F40.00 Without panic disorder

F40.01 With panic disorder

Includes: panic disorder with agoraphobia

F40.1   Social phobias

Social phobias often start in adolescence and are centred around a fear of scrutiny by other people in comparatively small groups (as opposed to crowds), usually leading to avoidance of social situations. Unlike most other phobias, social phobias are equally common in men and women. They may be discrete (i.e. restricted to eating in public, to public speaking, or to encounters with the opposite sex) or diffuse, involving almost all social situations outside the family circle. A fear of vomiting in public may be important. Direct eye-to-eye confrontation may be particularly stressful in some cultures. Social phobias are usually associated with low self-esteem and fear of criticism. They may present as a complaint of blushing, hand tremor, nausea, or urgency of micturition, the individual sometimes being convinced that one of these secondary manifestations of anxiety is the primary problem; symptoms may progress to panic attacks. Avoidance is often marked, and in extreme cases may result in almost complete social isolation.

Diagnostic guidelines
All of the following criteria should be fulfilled for a definite diagnosis:

(a)   the psychological, behavioural, or autonomic symptoms must be primarily manifestations of anxiety and not secondary to other symptoms such as delusions or obsessional thoughts;

(b)   the anxiety must be restricted to or predominate in particular social situations; and

(c)   the phobic situation is avoided whenever possible.

Includes: anthropophobia
          social neurosis

Differential diagnosis
Agoraphobia and depressive disorders are often prominent, and may both contribute to sufferers becoming 'housebound'. If the distinction between social phobia and agoraphobia is very difficult, precedence should be given to agoraphobia; a depressive diagnosis should not be made unless a full depressive syndrome can be identified clearly.

F40.2   *Specific (isolated) phobias*
These are phobias restricted to highly specific situations such as proximity to particular animals, heights, thunder, darkness, flying, closed spaces, urinating or defecating in public toilets, eating certain foods, dentistry, the sight of blood or injury, and the fear of exposure to specific diseases. Although the triggering situation is discrete, contact with it can evoke panic as in agoraphobia or social phobias. Specific phobias usually arise in childhood or early adult life and can persist for decades if they remain untreated. The seriousness of the resulting handicap depends on how easy it is for the sufferer to avoid the phobic situation. Fear of the phobic situation tends not to fluctuate, in contrast to agoraphobia. Radiation sickness and venereal infections and, more recently, AIDS are common subjects of disease phobias.

Diagnostic guidelines
All of the following should be fulfilled for a definite diagnosis:

(a)   the psychological or autonomic symptoms must be primary manifestations of anxiety, and not secondary to other symptoms such as delusion or obsessional thought;

(b)   the anxiety must be restricted to the presence of the particular phobic object or situation; and

One

(c) the phobic situation is avoided whenever possible.

Includes: acrophobia
animal phobias
claustrophobia
examination phobia
simple phobia

Differential diagnosis

It is usual for there to be no other psychiatric symptoms, in contrast to agoraphobia and social phobias. Blood-injury phobias differ from others in leading to bradycardia and sometimes syncope, rather than tachycardia. Fears of specific diseases such as cancer, heart disease, or venereal infection should be classified under hypochondriacal disorder (F45.2), unless they relate to specific situations where the disease might be acquired. If the conviction of disease reaches delusional intensity, the diagnosis should be delusional disorder (F22.0). Individuals who are convinced that they have an abnormality or disfigurement of a specific bodily (often facial) part, which is not objectively noticed by others (sometimes termed dysmorphophobia), should be classified under hypochondriacal disorder (F45.2) or delusional disorder (F22.0), depending upon the strength and persistence of their conviction.

F40.8 Other phobic anxiety disorders

F40.9 Phobic anxiety disorder, unspecified
Includes: phobia NOS
phobic states NOS

F41 Other anxiety disorders

Manifestations of anxiety are the major symptoms of these disorders and are not restricted to any particular environmental situation. Depressive and obsessional symptoms, and even some elements of phobic anxiety, may also be present, provided that they are clearly secondary or less severe.

F41.0 Panic disorder [episodic paroxysmal anxiety]

The essential features are recurrent attacks of severe anxiety (panic) which are not restricted to any particular situation or set of circumstances, and which are therefore unpredictable. As in other anxiety disorders, the dominant symptoms vary from person to person, but sudden onset of palpitations, chest pain, choking sensations, dizziness, and feelings of unreality (depersonalization or derealization) are common. There is also, almost invariably, a secondary fear of dying, losing control, or going mad. Individual attacks usually last for minutes only, though sometimes longer; their frequency and the course of the disorder are both rather variable. An individual in a panic attack often experiences a crescendo of fear and autonomic symptoms, which results in an exit, usually hurried, from wherever he or she may be. If this occurs in a specific situation, such as on a bus or in a crowd, the patient may subsequently avoid that situation. Similarly, frequent and unpredictable panic attacks produce fear of being alone or going into public places. A panic attack is often followed by a persistent fear of having another attack.

Diagnostic guidelines

In this classification, a panic attack that occurs in an established phobic situation is regarded as an expression of the severity of the phobia, which should be given diagnostic precedence. Panic disorder should be the main diagnosis only in the absence of any of the phobias in F40.–.

For a definite diagnosis, several severe attacks of autonomic anxiety should have occurred within a period of about 1 month:

(a)   in circumstances where there is no objective danger;
(b)   without being confined to known or predictable situations; and
(c)   with comparative freedom from anxiety symptoms between attacks (although anticipatory anxiety is common).

Includes: panic attack
             panic state

Differential diagnosis

Panic disorder must be distinguished from panic attacks occurring as part of established phobic disorders as already noted. Panic attacks may be secondary to depressive disorders, particularly in men, and if the criteria for a depressive disorder are fulfilled at the same time, the panic disorder should not be given as the main diagnosis.

F41.1   Generalized anxiety disorder

(In the ICD-10 diagnostic criteria for research, the diagnostic code for generalized anxiety disorder of childhood is listed under F93.8. However in the ICD-10, Clinical Descriptions and Diagnostic Guidelines, it is included under the general rubric General Anxiety

Disorder, F41.1. Whilst the diagnostic criteria for research in 93.8 do apply, the condition should be classified here in F41.1.)

The essential feature is excessive anxiety and worrying (apprehensive expectation), which is generalized and persistent but not restricted to, or even strongly predominating in, any particular environmental circumstances (i.e. it is 'free-floating'). As in other anxiety disorders the dominant symptoms are highly variable, but characteristic complaints include restlessness, being easily fatigued, difficulty concentrating, irritability, muscle tension, and disturbed sleep. Fears that the sufferer or a relative will shortly become ill or have an accident are often expressed, together with a variety of other worries and forebodings. The individual finds it difficult to control such worries and there is associated impairment in social functioning. The course of the disorder is variable but tends to be fluctuating and chronic.

Diagnostic guidelines

The sufferer must have primary symptoms of excessive anxiety and/or worrying most days for at least several weeks at a time, and usually for several months. These symptoms should usually involve elements of:

(a) apprehension (worries about future misfortunes, feeling 'on edge', difficulty in concentrating, etc.);
(b) motor tension (restless fidgeting, tension headaches, trembling, inability to relax);
(c) fatigue (feeling tired or 'worn out');
(d) poor concentration (difficulty concentrating or mind going blank);
(e) irritability; and
(f) sleep disturbance (difficulty in falling or staying asleep, or restless, unsatisfying sleep)

The transient appearance (for a few days at a time) of other symptoms, particularly depression, does not rule out generalized anxiety disorder as a main diagnosis, but the sufferer must not meet the full criteria for depressive episode (F32.–), phobic anxiety disorder (F40.–), panic disorder (F41.0), or obsessive-compulsive disorder (F42.–)

Includes: anxiety neurosis
anxiety reaction
anxiety state
overanxious disorder of childhood
Excludes: neurasthenia (F48.0)

F41.2   Mixed anxiety and depressive disorder

This mixed category should be used when symptoms of both anxiety and depression are present, but neither set of symptoms, considered separately, is sufficiently severe to justify a diagnosis. If severe anxiety is present with a lesser degree of depression, one of the other categories for anxiety or phobic disorders should be used. When both depressive and anxiety syndromes are present and severe enough to justify individual diagnoses, both disorders should be recorded and this category should not be used; if, for practical reasons of recording, only one diagnosis can be made, depression should be given precedence. Some autonomic symptoms (tremor, palpitations, dry mouth, stomach churning, etc.) must be present, even if only intermittently; if only worry or over-concern is present, without autonomic symptoms, this category should not be used. If symptoms that fulfil the criteria for this disorder occur in close association with significant life changes or stressful life events, category F43.2, adjustment disorders, should be used.

Individuals with this mixture of comparatively mild symptoms are frequently seen in primary care, but many more cases exist among the population at large that never come to medical or psychiatric attention.

Includes: anxiety depression (mild or not persistent)
Excludes: persistent anxiety depression (dysthymia) (F34.1)

F41.3   Other mixed anxiety disorders

This category should be used for disorders that meet the criteria for generalized anxiety disorder (F41.1) and that also have prominent (although often short-lasting) features of other disorders in F40–F49, although the full criteria for these additional disorders are not met. The commonest examples are obsessive-compulsive disorder (F42.–), dissociative disorders (F44.–), somatization disorder (F45.0), undifferentiated somatoform disorder (F45.1), and hypochondriacal disorder (F45.2). If symptoms that fulfil the criteria for this disorder occur in close association with significant life changes or stressful life events, category F43.2, adjustment disorders, should be used.

F41.8   Other specified anxiety disorders
Includes: anxiety hysteria

F41.9   Anxiety disorder, unspecified
Includes: anxiety NOS

One

F42 Obsessive-compulsive disorder

The essential feature of this disorder is recurrent obsessional thoughts or compulsive acts. (For brevity, 'obsessional' will be used subsequently in place of 'obsessive-compulsive' when referring to symptoms.) Obsessional thoughts are ideas, images or impulses that enter the individual's mind again and again in a stereotyped form. They are almost invariably distressing (because they are violent or obscene, or simply because they are perceived as senseless) and the sufferer often tries, unsuccessfully, to resist them. They are, however, recognized as the individual's own thoughts, even though they are involuntary and often repugnant. Compulsive acts or rituals are stereotyped behaviours that are repeated again and again. They are not inherently enjoyable, nor do they result in the completion of inherently useful tasks. The individual often views them as preventing some objectively unlikely event, often involving harm to or caused by himself or herself. Usually, though not invariably, this behaviour is recognized by the individual as pointless or ineffectual and repeated attempts are made to resist it; in very long-standing cases, resistance may be minimal. Autonomic anxiety symptoms are often present, but distressing feelings of internal or psychic tension without obvious autonomic arousal are also common. There is a close relationship between obsessional symptoms, particularly obsessional thoughts, and depression. Individuals with obsessive-compulsive disorder often have depressive symptoms, and patients suffering from recurrent depressive disorder (F33.–) may develop obsessional thoughts during their episodes of depression. In either situation, increases or decreases in the severity of the depressive symptoms are generally accompanied by parallel changes in the severity of the obsessional symptoms.

Obsessive-compulsive disorder is equally common in men and women, and there are often prominent anankastic features in the underlying personality. Onset is usually in childhood or early adult life. The course is variable and more likely to be chronic in the absence of significant depressive symptoms.

Diagnostic guidelines

For a definite diagnosis, obsessional symptoms or compulsive acts, or both, must be present on most days for at least 2 successive weeks and be a source of distress or interference with activities. The obsessional symptoms should have the following characteristics:

(a)   they must be recognized as the individual's own thoughts or impulses;
(b)   there must be at least one thought or act that is still resisted unsuccess-fully, even though others may be present which the sufferer no longer resists;
(c)   the thought of carrying out the act must not in itself be pleasurable (sim-ple relief of tension or anxiety is not regarded as pleasure in this sense);
(d)   the thoughts, images, or impulses must be unpleasantly repetitive.

> *Includes*: anankastic neurosis
>   obsessional neurosis
>   obsessive-compulsive neurosis

Differential diagnosis

Differentiating between obsessive-compulsive disorder and a depressive disorder may be difficult because these two types of symptoms so fre-quently occur together. In an acute episode of disorder, precedence should be given to the symptoms that developed first; when both types are present but neither predominates, it is usually best to regard the depression as primary. In chronic disorders the symptoms that most fre-quently persist in the absence of the other should be given priority.

Occasional panic attacks or mild phobic symptoms are no bar to the diagnosis. However, obsessional symptoms developing in the presence of schizophrenia, Tourette's syndrome, or organic mental disorder should be regarded as part of these conditions.

Although obsessional thoughts and compulsive acts commonly coex-ist, it is useful to be able to specify one set of symptoms as predominant in some individuals, since they may respond to different treatments.

F42.0   Predominantly obsessional thoughts or ruminations

These may take the form of ideas, mental images, or impulses to act. They are very variable in content but nearly always distressing to the individual. Sometimes the ideas are merely futile, involving an endless and quasi-philosophical consideration of imponderable alternatives. This indecisive consideration of alternatives is an important element in many other obsessional ruminations and is often associated with an inability to make trivial but necessary decisions in day-to-day living.

The relationship between obsessional ruminations and depression is particularly close: a diagnosis of obsessive-compulsive disorder should be preferred only if ruminations arise or persist in the absence of a depressive disorder.

F42.1   *Predominantly compulsive acts [obsessional rituals]*

The majority of compulsive acts are concerned with cleaning (particularly hand-washing), repeated checking to ensure that a potentially dangerous situation has not been allowed to develop, or orderliness and tidiness. Underlying the overt behaviour is a fear, usually of danger either to or caused by the patient, and the ritual act is an ineffectual or symbolic attempt to avert that danger. Compulsive ritual acts may occupy many hours every day and are sometimes associated with marked indecisiveness and slowness. Overall, they are equally common in the two sexes but hand-washing rituals are more common in women and slowness without repetition is more common in men.

Compulsive ritual acts are less closely associated with depression than obsessional thoughts and are more readily amenable to behavioural therapies.

F42.2   *Mixed obsessional thoughts and acts*

Most obsessive-compulsive individuals have elements of both obsessional thinking and compulsive behaviour. This subcategory should be used if the two are equally prominent, as is often the case, but it is useful to specify only one if it is clearly predominant, since thoughts and acts may respond to different treatments.

F42.8   *Other obsessive-compulsive disorders*

F42.9   *Obsessive-compulsive disorder, unspecified*

F43   Reaction to severe stress, and adjustment disorders

This category differs from others in that it includes disorders identifiable not only on grounds of symptomatology and course but also on the basis of one or other of two causative influences – an exceptionally stressful life event producing an acute stress reaction, or a significant life change leading to continued unpleasant circumstances that result in an adjustment disorder. Less severe psychosocial stress ('life events') may precipitate the onset or contribute to the presentation of a very wide range of disorders classified elsewhere in this work, but the etiological importance of such stress is not always clear and in each case will be found to depend on individual, often idiosyncratic, vulnerability. In other words, the stress is neither necessary nor sufficient to explain the occurrence and form of the disorder. In contrast, the disorders brought together in this category are thought to arise always as a direct consequence of the acute severe stress or continued trauma. The stressful event or the continuing unpleasantness of circumstances is the primary and overriding causal factor, and the disorder would not have occurred without its impact. Reactions to severe stress and adjustment disorders in all age groups are included in this category.

Although each individual symptom of which both the acute stress reaction and the adjustment disorder are composed may occur in other disorders, there are some special features in the way the symptoms are manifest that justify the inclusion of these states as a clinical entity. The third condition in this section – post-traumatic stress disorder – has relatively specific and characteristic clinical features.

These disorders can thus be regarded as maladaptive responses to severe or continued stress, in that they interfere with successful coping mechanisms and thus lead to problems in social functioning.

F43.0   *Acute stress reaction*

A transient disorder of significant severity that develops in an individual without any other apparent mental disorder in response to exceptional physical and/or mental stress and which usually subsides within hours or days. The stressor may be an overwhelming traumatic experience involving serious threat to the security or physical integrity of the individual or of a loved person(s) (e.g. natural catastrophe, accident, battle, criminal assault, rape), or an unusually sudden and threatening change in the social position and/or network of the individual, such as multiple bereavement or domestic fire. The risk of this disorder developing is increased if physical exhaustion or organic factors are also present.

Individual vulnerability and coping capacity play a role in the occurrence and severity of acute stress reactions, as evidenced by the fact that not all people exposed to exceptional stress develop the disorder. The symptoms show great variation but typically they include an initial state of 'daze', with some constriction of the field of consciousness and narrowing of attention, inability to comprehend stimuli, and disorientation. This state may be followed either by further withdrawal from the surrounding situation (to the extent of a dissociative stupor – see F44.2), or by agitation and over-activity (flight reaction or fugue). Autonomic signs of panic anxiety (tachycardia, sweating, flushing) are commonly present. The symptoms usually appear within minutes of the impact of the stressful stimulus or event, and disappear within 2–3 days (often within hours). Partial or complete amnesia (see F44.0) for the episode may be present.

Diagnostic guidelines

There must be an immediate and clear temporal connection between the impact of an exceptional stressor and the onset of symptoms; onset is usually within a few minutes, if not immediate. In addition, the symptoms:

(a) show a mixed and usually changing picture; in addition to the initial state of 'daze', depression, anxiety, anger, despair, overactivity, and withdrawal may all be seen, but no one type of symptom predominates for long;

(b) resolve rapidly (within a few hours at the most) in those cases where removal from the stressful environment is possible; in cases where the stress continues or cannot by its nature be reversed, the symptoms usually begin to diminish after 24–48 hours and are usually minimal after about 3 days.

This diagnosis should not be used to cover sudden exacerbations of symptoms in individuals already showing symptoms that fulfil the criteria of any other psychiatric disorder, except for those in F60.– (personality disorders). However, a history of previous psychiatric disorder does not invalidate the use of this diagnosis.

Includes: acute crisis reaction
combat fatigue
crisis state
psychic shock

F43.1 *Post-traumatic stress disorder*

This arises as a delayed and/or protracted response to a stressful event or situation (either short- or long-lasting) of an exceptionally threatening or catastrophic nature, which is likely to cause pervasive distress in almost anyone (e.g. natural or man-made disaster, combat, serious accident, witnessing the violent death of others, or being the victim of torture, terrorism, rape, or other crime). Predisposing factors such as personality traits (e.g. compulsive, asthenic) or previous history of neurotic illness may lower the threshold for the development of the syndrome or aggravate its course, but they are neither necessary nor sufficient to explain its occurrence.

Typical symptoms include episodes of repeated reliving of the trauma in intrusive memories ('flashbacks') or dreams, occurring against the persisting background of a sense of 'numbness' and emotional blunting, detachment from other people, unresponsiveness to surroundings, anhedonia, and avoidance of activities and situations reminiscent of the trauma. Commonly there is fear and avoidance of cues that remind the sufferer of the original trauma. Rarely, there may be dramatic, acute bursts of fear, panic or aggression, triggered by stimuli arousing a sudden recollection and/or re-enactment of the trauma or of the original reaction to it.

There is usually a state of autonomic hyperarousal with hypervigilance, an enhanced startle reaction, and insomnia. Anxiety and depression are commonly associated with the above symptoms and signs, and suicidal ideation is not infrequent. Excessive use of alcohol or drugs may be a complicating factor.

The onset follows the trauma with a latency period that may range from a few weeks to months (but rarely exceeds 6 months). The course is fluctuating but recovery can be expected in the majority of cases. In a small proportion of patients the condition may show a chronic course over many years and a transition to an enduring personality change (see F62.0).

Diagnostic guidelines

This disorder should not generally be diagnosed unless there is evidence that it arose within 6 months of a traumatic event of exceptional severity. A 'probable' diagnosis might still be possible if the delay between the event and the onset was longer than 6 months, provided that the clinical manifestations are typical and no alternative identification of the disorder (e.g. as an anxiety or obsessive-compulsive disorder or depressive episode) is plausible. In addition to evidence of trauma, there must be a repetitive, intrusive recollection or re-enactment of the event in memories, daytime imagery, or dreams. Conspicuous emotional detachment, numbing of feeling, and avoidance of stimuli that might arouse recollection of the trauma are often present but are not essential for the diagnosis. The autonomic disturbances, mood disorder, and behavioural abnormalities all contribute to the diagnosis but are not of prime importance.

Includes: traumatic neurosis

F43.2   Adjustment disorders

States of subjective distress and emotional disturbance, usually interfering with social functioning and performance, and arising in the period of adaptation to a significant life change or to the consequences of a stressful life event (including the presence or possibility of serious physical

One

illness). The stressor may have affected the integrity of an individual's social network (through bereavement or separation experiences) or the wider system of social supports and values (migration or refugee status). The stressor may involve only the individual or also his or her group or community.

Individual predisposition or vulnerability plays a greater role in the risk of occurrence and the shaping of the manifestations of adjustment disorders than it does in the other conditions in F43.–, but it is nevertheless assumed that the condition would not have arisen without the stressor. The manifestations vary, and include depressed mood, anxiety, worry (or a mixture of these), a feeling of inability to cope, plan ahead, or continue in the present situation, and some degree of disability in the performance of daily routine. The individual may feel liable to dramatic behaviour or outbursts of violence, but these rarely occur. However, conduct disorders (e.g. aggressive or dissocial behaviour) may be an associated feature, particularly in adolescents. None of the symptoms is of sufficient severity or prominence in its own right to justify a more specific diagnosis. In children, regressive phenomena such as return to bed-wetting, babyish speech, or thumb-sucking are frequently part of the symptom pattern. If these features predominate, F43.23 should be used.

The onset is usually within 1 month of the occurrence of the stressful event or life change, and the duration of symptoms does not usually exceed 6 months, except in the case of prolonged depressive reaction (F43.21). If the symptoms persist beyond this period, the diagnosis should be changed according to the clinical picture present, and any continuing stress can be coded in Axis Five.

Grief reactions of any duration, considered to be abnormal because of their form or content, should be coded as F43.22, F43.23, F43.24 or F43.25, and those that are still intense and last longer than 6 months as F43.21 (prolonged depressive reaction).

Diagnostic guidelines
Diagnosis depends on a careful evaluation of the relationship between:

(a)   form, content, and severity of symptoms;
(b)   previous history and personality; and
(c)   stressful event, situation, or life crisis.

The presence of this third factor should be clearly established and there should be strong, though perhaps presumptive, evidence that the disorder would not have arisen without it. If the stressor is relatively minor, or if a temporal connection (less than 3 months) cannot be demonstrated, the disorder should be classified elsewhere, according to its presenting features.

Includes: culture shock
              grief reaction
              hospitalism in children
Excludes: separation anxiety disorder of childhood (F93.0)

If the criteria for adjustment disorder are satisfied, the clinical form or predominant features can be specified by a fifth character:

F43.20 Brief depressive reaction
A transient, mild depressive state of duration not exceeding 1 month.

F43.21 Prolonged depressive reaction
A mild depressive state occurring in response to a prolonged exposure to a stressful situation but of duration not exceeding 2 years.

F43.22 Mixed anxiety and depressive reaction
Both anxiety and depressive symptoms are prominent, but at levels no greater than specified in mixed anxiety and depressive disorder (F41.2) or other mixed anxiety disorder (F41.3).

F43.23 With predominant disturbance of other emotions
The symptoms are usually of several types of emotion, such as anxiety, depression, worry, tensions, and anger. Symptoms of anxiety and depression may fulfil the criteria for mixed anxiety and depressive disorder (F41.2) or other mixed anxiety disorder (F41.3), but they are not so predominant that other more specific depressive or anxiety disorders can be diagnosed. This category should be used for reactions in children in which regressive behaviour such as bed-wetting or thumb-sucking are also present.

F43.24 With predominant disturbance of conduct
The main disturbance is one involving conduct, e.g. an adolescent grief reaction resulting in aggressive or dissocial behaviour.

F43.25 With mixed disturbance of emotions and conduct
Both emotional symptoms and disturbance of conduct are prominent features.

F43.28 With other specified predominant symptoms

F43.8   Other reactions to severe stress

F43.9   Reaction to severe stress, unspecified

F44   Dissociative [conversion] disorders

The common theme shared by dissociative (or conversion) disorders is a partial or complete loss of the normal integration between memories of the past, awareness of identity and immediate sensations, and control of bodily movements. There is normally a considerable degree of conscious control over the memories and sensations that can be selected for immediate attention, and the movements that are to be carried out. In the dissociative disorders it is presumed that this ability to exercise a conscious and selective control is impaired, to a degree that can vary from day to day or even from hour to hour. It is usually very difficult to assess the extent to which some of the loss of functions might be under voluntary control.

These disorders have previously been classified as various types of 'conversion hysteria', but it now seems best to avoid the term 'hysteria' as far as possible, in view of its many and varied meanings. Dissociative disorders as described here are presumed to be 'psychogenic' in origin, being associated closely in time with traumatic events, insoluble and intolerable problems, or disturbed relationships. It is therefore often possible to make interpretations and presumptions about the individual's means of dealing with intolerable stress, but concepts derived from any one particular theory, such as 'unconscious motivation' and 'secondary gain', are not included among the guidelines or criteria for diagnosis.

The term 'conversion' is widely applied to some of these disorders, and implies that the unpleasant affect, engendered by the problems and conflicts that the individual cannot solve, is somehow transformed into the symptoms.

The onset and termination of dissociative states are often reported as being sudden, but they are rarely observed except during contrived interactions or procedures such as hypnosis or abreaction. Change in or disappearance of a dissociative state may be limited to the duration of such procedures. All types of dissociative state tend to remit after a few weeks or months, particularly if their onset was associated with a traumatic life event. More chronic states, particularly paralyses and anæsthesias, may develop (sometimes more slowly) if they are associated with insoluble problems or interpersonal difficulties. Dissociative states that have endured for more than 1–2 years before coming to psychiatric attention are often resistant to therapy.

Individuals with dissociative disorders often show a striking denial of problems or difficulties that may be obvious to others. Any problems that they themselves recognize may be attributed by patients to the dissociative symptoms.

Depersonalization and derealization are *not* included here, since in these syndromes only limited aspects of personal identity are usually affected, and there is no associated loss of performance in terms of sensations, memories, or movements.

Diagnostic guidelines
For a definite diagnosis the following should be present:

(a) the clinical features as specified for the individual disorders in F44.–;
(b) no evidence of a physical disorder that might explain the symptoms;
(c) evidence for psychological causation, in the form of clear association in time with stressful events and problems or disturbed relationships (even if denied by the individual).

Convincing evidence of psychological causation may be difficult to find, even though strongly suspected. In the presence of known disorders of the central or peripheral nervous system, the diagnosis of dissociative disorder should be made with great caution. In the absence of evidence for psychological causation, the diagnosis should remain provisional, and enquiry into both physical and psychological aspects should continue.

Includes: conversion hysteria
conversion reaction
hysteria
hysterical psychosis
Excludes: malingering [conscious simulation] (Z76.5)

F44.0   Dissociative amnesia
The main feature is loss of memory, usually of important recent events, which is not due to organic mental disorder and is too extensive to be explained by ordinary forgetfulness or fatigue. The amnesia is usually centred on traumatic events, such as accidents or unexpected bereavements, and is usually partial and selective. The extent and completeness

of the amnesia often vary from day to day and between investigators, but there is a persistent common core that cannot be recalled in the waking state. Complete and generalized amnesia is rare; it is usually part of a fugue (F44.1) and, if so, should be classified as such.

The affective states that accompany amnesia are very varied, but severe depression is rare. Perplexity, distress, and varying degrees of attention-seeking behaviour may be evident, but calm acceptance is also sometimes striking. Purposeless local wandering may occur; it is usually accompanied by self-neglect and rarely lasts more than a day or two.

Diagnostic guidelines
A definite diagnosis requires:

(a) amnesia, either partial or complete, for recent events that are of a trau-matic or stressful nature (these aspects may emerge only when other informants are available);

(b) absence of organic brain disorders, intoxication, or excessive fatigue.

Differential diagnosis
In organic mental disorders, there are usually other signs of disturbance in the nervous system, plus obvious and consistent signs of clouding of consciousness, disorientation, and fluctuating awareness. Loss of very recent memory is more typical of organic states, irrespective of any pos-sibly traumatic events or problems. 'Blackouts' due to abuse of alcohol or drugs are closely associated with the time of abuse, and the lost mem-ories can never be regained. The short-term memory loss of the amnesic state (Korsakov's syndrome), in which immediate recall is normal but recall after only 2–3 minutes is lost, is not found in dissociative amnesia.

Amnesia following concussion or serious head injury is usually retro-grade, although in severe cases it may be anterograde also; dissociative amnesia is usually predominantly retrograde. Only dissociative amnesia can be modified by hypnosis or abreaction. Postictal amnesia in epilep-tics, and other states of stupor or mutism occasionally found in schizo-phrenic or depressive illnesses, can usually be differentiated by other characteristics of the underlying illness.

The most difficult differentiation is from conscious simulation of amnesia (malingering), and repeated and detailed assessment of premor-bid personality and motivation may be required.

Excludes: alcohol- or other psychoactive substance-induced amnesic disorder (F10–F19 with common fourth character .x6)
amnesia NOS (R41.3)

anterograde amnesia (R41.1)
nonalcoholic organic amnesic syndrome (F04)
postictal amnesia in epilepsy (G40.–)
retrograde amnesia (R41.2)

F44.1   Dissociative fugue

Dissociative fugue has all the features of dissociative amnesia, plus an apparently purposeful journey away from home or place of work during which self-care is maintained. In some cases, a new identity may be assumed, usually only for a few days but occasionally for long periods of time and to a surprising degree of completeness. Organized travel may be to places previously known and of emotional significance. Although there is amnesia for the period of the fugue, the individual's behaviour during this time may appear completely normal to independent observers.

Diagnostic guidelines

For a definite diagnosis there should be:

(a) the features of dissociative amnesia (F44.0);
(b) purposeful travel beyond the usual everyday range (the differentiation between travel and wandering must be made by those with local knowledge); and
(c) maintenance of basic self-care (eating, washing, etc.) and simple social interaction with strangers (such as buying tickets or petrol, asking directions, ordering meals).

Differential diagnosis

Differentiation from postictal fugue, seen particularly after temporal lobe epilepsy, is usually clear because of the history of epilepsy, the lack of stressful events or problems, and the less purposeful and more fragmented activities and travel of the epileptic.

As with dissociative amnesia, differentiation from conscious simulation of a fugue may be very difficult.

F44.2   Dissociative stupor

The individual's behaviour fulfils the criteria for stupor, but examination and investigation reveal no evidence of a physical cause. In addition, as in other dissociative disorders, there is positive evidence of psychogenic causation in the form of either recent stressful events or prominent interpersonal or social problems.

Stupor is diagnosed on the basis of a profound diminution or absence of voluntary movement and normal responsiveness to external stimuli such as light, noise, and touch. The individual lies or sits largely motionless for long periods of time. Speech and spontaneous and purposeful movement are completely or almost completely absent. Although some degree of disturbance of consciousness may be present, muscle tone, posture, breathing, and sometimes eye-opening and coordinated eye movements are such that it is clear that the individual is neither asleep nor unconscious.

Diagnostic guidelines

For a definite diagnosis there should be:

(a)   stupor, as described above;
(b)   absence of a physical or other psychiatric disorder that might explain the stupor; and
(c)   evidence of recent stressful events or current problems.

Differential diagnosis

Dissociative stupor must be differentiated from catatonic stupor and depressive or manic stupor. The stupor of catatonic schizophrenia is often preceded by symptoms or behaviour suggestive of schizophrenia. Depressive and manic stupor usually develop comparatively slowly, so a history from another informant should be decisive. Both depressive and manic stupor are increasingly rare in many countries as early treatment of affective illness becomes more widespread.

F44.3   Trance and possession disorders

Disorders in which there is a temporary loss of both the sense of personal identity and full awareness of the surroundings; in some instances the individual acts as if taken over by another personality, spirit, deity, or 'force'. Attention and awareness may be limited to or concentrated upon only one or two aspects of the immediate environment, and there is often a limited but repeated set of movements, postures, and utterances. Only trance disorders that are involuntary or unwanted, and that intrude into ordinary activities by occurring outside (or being a prolongation of) religious or other culturally accepted situations should be included here.

Trance disorders occurring during the course of schizophrenic or acute psychoses with hallucinations or delusions, or multiple personality should not be included here, nor should this category be used if the trance disorder is judged to be closely associated with any physical disorder (such as temporal lobe epilepsy or head injury) or with psychoactive substance intoxication.

F44.4–F44.7 *Dissociative disorders of movement and sensation*

In these disorders there is a loss of or interference with movements or loss of sensations (usually cutaneous). The patient therefore presents as having a physical disorder, although none can be found that would explain the symptoms. The symptoms can often be seen to represent the patient's concept of physical disorder, which may be at variance with physiological or anatomical principles. In addition, assessment of the patient's mental state and social situation usually suggests that the disability resulting from the loss of functions is helping the patient to escape from an unpleasant conflict, or to express dependency or resentment indirectly. Although problems or conflicts may be evident to others, the patient often denies their presence and attributes any distress to the symptoms or the resulting disability.

The degree of disability resulting from all these types of symptom may vary from occasion to occasion, depending upon the number and type of other people present, and upon the emotional state of the patient. In other words, a variable amount of attention-seeking behaviour may be present in addition to a central and unvarying core of loss of movement or sensation that is not under voluntary control.

In some patients, the symptoms usually develop in close relationship to psychological stress, but in others this link does not emerge. Calm acceptance (*belle indifférence*) of serious disability may be striking, but is not universal; it is also found in well-adjusted individuals facing obvious and serious physical illness.

Premorbid abnormalities of personal relationships and personality are usually found, and close relatives and friends may have suffered from physical illness with symptoms resembling those of the patient. Mild and transient varieties of these disorders are often seen in adolescence, particularly in girls, but the chronic varieties are usually found in young adults. A few individuals establish a repetitive pattern of reaction to stress by the production of these disorders, and may still manifest this later in life.

Disorders involving only *loss* of sensations are included here; disorders involving additional sensations such as pain, and other complex sensations mediated by the autonomic nervous system are included in somatoform disorders (F45.–).

One

Diagnostic guidelines

The diagnosis should be made with great caution in the presence of physical disorders of the nervous system, or in a previously well-adjusted individual with normal family and social relationships.

For a definite diagnosis:

(a) there should be no evidence of physical disorder; and

(b) sufficient must be known about the psychological and social setting and personal relationships of the patient to allow a convincing formulation to be made of the reasons for the appearance of the disorder.

The diagnosis should remain probable or provisional if there is any doubt about the contribution of actual or possible physical disorders, or if it is impossible to achieve an understanding of why the disorder has developed. In cases that are puzzling or not clear-cut, the possibility of the later appearance of serious physical or psychiatric disorders should always be kept in mind.

Differential diagnosis

The early stages of progressive neurological disorders, particularly multiple sclerosis and systemic lupus erythematosus, may be confused with dissociative disorders of movement and sensation. Patients reacting to early multiple sclerosis with distress and attention-seeking behaviour pose especially difficult problems; comparatively long periods of assessment and observation may be needed before the diagnostic probabilities become clear.

Multiple and ill-defined somatic complaints should be classified elsewhere, under somatoform disorders (F45.–) or neurasthenia (F48.0).

Isolated dissociative symptoms may occur during major mental disorders such as schizophrenia or severe depression, but these disorders are usually obvious and should take precedence over the dissociative symptoms for diagnostic and coding purposes.

Conscious simulation of loss of movement and sensation is often very difficult to distinguish from dissociation; the decision will rest upon detailed observation, and upon obtaining an understanding of the personality of the patient, the circumstances surrounding the onset of the disorder, and the consequences of recovery versus continued disability.

F44.4 Dissociative motor disorders

The commonest varieties of dissociative motor disorder are loss of ability to move the whole or a part of a limb or limbs. Paralysis may be partial, with movements being weak or slow, or complete. Various forms and variable degrees of incoordination (ataxia) may be evident, particularly in the legs, resulting in bizarre gait or inability to stand unaided (astasia-abasia). There may also be exaggerated trembling or shaking of one or more extremities or the whole body. There may be close resemblance to almost any variety of ataxia, apraxia, akinesia, aphonia, dysarthria, dyskinesia, or paralysis.

Includes: psychogenic aphonia
psychogenic dysphonia

F44.5   *Dissociative convulsions*
Dissociative convulsions (pseudoseizures) may mimic epileptic seizures very closely in terms of movements, but tongue-biting, serious bruising due to falling, and incontinence of urine are rare in dissociative convulsion, and loss of consciousness is absent or replaced by a state of stupor or trance.

F44.6   *Dissociative anaesthesia and sensory loss*
Anaesthetic areas of skin often have boundaries that make it clear that they are associated more with the patient's ideas about bodily functions than with medical knowledge. There may also be differential loss between the sensory modalities that cannot be due to a neurological lesion. Sensory loss may be accompanied by complaints of paraesthesia.

Loss of vision is rarely total in dissociative disorders, and visual disturbances are more often a loss of acuity, general blurring of vision, or 'tunnel vision'. In spite of complaints of visual loss, the patient's general mobility and motor performance are often surprisingly well preserved.

Dissociative deafness and anosmia are far less common than loss of sensation or vision.

Includes: psychogenic deafness

F44.7   *Mixed dissociative [conversion] disorders*
Mixtures of the disorders specified above (F44.0–F44.6) should be coded here.

F44.8   *Other dissociative [conversion] disorders*

F44.80 Ganser's syndrome
The complex disorder described by Ganser, which is characterized by

One

'approximate answers', usually accompanied by several other dissociative symptoms, often in circumstances that suggest a psychogenic etiology, should be coded here.

F44.81 Multiple personality disorder
This disorder is rare, and controversy exists about the extent to which it is iatrogenic or culture-specific. The essential feature is the apparent existence of two or more distinct personalities within an individual, with only one of them being evident at a time. Each personality is complete, with its own memories, behaviour, and preferences; these may be in marked contrast to the single premorbid personality.

In the common form with two personalities, one personality is usually dominant but neither has access to the memories of the other and the two are almost always unaware of each other's existence. Change from one personality to another in the first instance is usually sudden and closely associated with traumatic events. Subsequent changes are often limited to dramatic or stressful events, or occur during sessions with a therapist that involve relaxation, hypnosis, or abreaction.

F44.82 Transient dissociative [conversion] disorders occurring in childhood and adolescence

F44.88 Other specified dissociative [conversion] disorders

Includes: psychogenic confusion
twilight state

F44.9   Dissociative [conversion] disorder, unspecified

F45   Somatoform disorders

The main feature of somatoform disorders is repeated presentation of physical symptoms, together with persistent requests for medical investigations, in spite of repeated negative findings and reassurances by doctors that the symptoms have no physical basis. If any physical disorders are present, they do not explain the nature and extent of the symptoms or the distress and preoccupation of the patient. Even when the onset and continuation of the symptoms bear a close relationship with unpleasant life events or with difficulties or conflicts, the patient usually resists attempts to discuss the possibility of psychological causation; this may even be the case in the presence of obvious depressive and anxiety symptoms. The degree of understanding, either physical or psychologi-cal, that can be achieved about the cause of the symptoms is often disap-pointing and frustrating for both patient and doctor.

In these disorders there is often a degree of attention-seeking (histri-onic) behaviour, particularly in patients who are resentful of their failure to persuade doctors of the essentially physical nature of their illness and of the need for further investigations or examinations.

Differential diagnosis

Differentiation from hypochondriacal delusions usually depends upon close acquaintance with the patient. Although the beliefs are long-stand-ing and appear to be held against reason, the degree of conviction is usually susceptible, to some degree and in the short term, to argument, reassurance, and the performance of yet another examination or investigation. In addition, the presence of unpleasant and frightening physical sensations can be regarded as a culturally acceptable explana-tion for the development and persistence of a conviction of physical ill-ness.

Excludes: dissociative disorders (F44.–)
hair-plucking (F98.4)
lalling (F80.0)
lisping (F80.8)
nail-biting (F98.8)
psychological or behavioural factors associated with disorders or diseases classified elsewhere (F54)
sexual dysfunction, not caused by organic disorder or disease (F52.–)
thumb-sucking (F98.8)
tic disorders (in childhood and adolescence) (F95.–)
Tourette's syndrome (F95.2)
trichotillomania (F63.3)

F45.0   Somatization disorder

The main features are multiple, recurrent, and frequently changing phys-ical symptoms, which have usually been present for several years before the patient is referred to a psychiatrist. Most patients have a long and complicated history of contact with both primary and specialist medical services, during which many negative investigations or fruitless opera-tions may have been carried out. Symptoms may be referred to any part or system of the body, but gastrointestinal sensations (pain, belching,

One

regurgitation, vomiting, nausea, etc.), and abnormal skin sensations (itching, burning, tingling, numbness, soreness, etc.) and blotchiness are among the commonest. Sexual and menstrual complaints are also common.

Marked depression and anxiety are frequently present and may justify specific treatment.

The course of the disorder is chronic and fluctuating, and is often associated with long-standing disruption of social, interpersonal, and family behaviour. The disorder is far more common in women than in men, and usually starts in early adult life but may be seen in adolescence.

Dependence upon or abuse of medication (usually sedatives and analgesics) often results from the frequent courses of medication.

Diagnostic guidelines
A definite diagnosis requires the presence of all of the following:

(a) at least 2 years of multiple and variable physical symptoms for which no adequate physical explanation has been found;

(b) persistent refusal to accept the advice or reassurance of several doctors that there is no physical explanation for the symptoms;

(c) some degree of impairment of social and family functioning attributable to the nature of the symptoms and resulting behaviour.

Includes: multiple complaint syndrome
multiple psychosomatic disorder

Differential diagnosis
In diagnosis, differentiation from the following disorders is essential:

Physical disorders
Patients with long-standing somatization disorder have the same chance of developing independent physical disorders as any other person of their age, and further investigations or consultations should be considered if there is a shift in the emphasis or stability of the physical complaints which suggests possible physical disease.

Affective (depressive) and anxiety disorders
Varying degrees of depression and anxiety commonly accompany somatization disorders, but need not be specified separately unless they are sufficiently marked and persistent as to justify a diagnosis in their own

right. The onset of multiple somatic symptoms after the age of 40 years may be an early manifestation of a primarily depressive disorder.

Hypochondriacal disorder

In somatization disorders, the emphasis is on the symptoms themselves and their individual effects, whereas in hypochondriacal disorder, attention is directed more to the presence of an underlying progressive and serious disease process and its disabling consequences. In hypochondriacal disorder, the patient tends to ask for investigations to determine or confirm the nature of the underlying disease, whereas the patient with somatization disorder asks for treatment to remove the symptoms. In somatization disorder there is usually excessive drug use, together with noncompliance over long periods, whereas patients with hypochondriacal disorder fear drugs and their side-effects, and seek for reassurance by frequent visits to different physicians.

Delusional disorders

(such as schizophrenia with somatic delusions, and depressive disorders with hypochondriacal delusions). The bizarre qualities of the beliefs, together with fewer physical symptoms of more constant nature, are most typical of the delusional disorders.

Short-lived (e.g. less than 2 years) and less striking symptom patterns are better classified as undifferentiated somatoform disorder (F45.1).

F45.1   Undifferentiated somatoform disorder

When physical complaints are multiple, varying and persistent, but the complete and typical clinical picture of somatization disorder is not fulfilled, this category should be considered. For instance, the forceful and dramatic manner of complaint may be lacking, the complaints may be comparatively few in number, or the associated impairment of social and family functioning may be totally absent. There may or may not be grounds for presuming a psychological causation, but there must be no physical basis for the symptoms upon which the psychiatric diagnosis is based.

If a distinct possibility of underlying physical disorder still exists, or if the psychiatric assessment is not completed at the time of diagnostic coding, other categories from the relevant chapters of ICD-10 should be used.
Includes: undifferentiated psychosomatic disorder

Differential diagnosis

As for the full syndrome of somatization disorder (F45.0).

F45.2   Hypochondriacal disorder

The essential feature is a persistent preoccupation with the possibility of having one or more serious and progressive physical disorders. Patients manifest persistent somatic complaints or persistent preoccupation with their physical appearance. Normal or commonplace sensations and appearances are often interpreted by a patient as abnormal and distressing, and attention is usually focused on only one or two organs or systems of the body. The feared physical disorder or disfigurement may be named by the patient, but even so the degree of conviction about its presence and the emphasis upon one disorder rather than another usually varies between consultations; the patient will usually entertain the possibility that other or additional physical disorders may exist in addition to the one given pre-eminence.

Marked depression and anxiety are often present, and may justify additional diagnosis. The disorders rarely present for the first time after the age of 50 years, and the course of both symptoms and disability is usually chronic and fluctuating. There must be no fixed delusions about bodily functions or shape. Fears of the presence of one or more diseases (nosophobia) should be classified here.

This syndrome occurs in both men and women, and there are no special familial characteristics (in contrast to somatization disorder).

Many individuals, especially those with milder forms of the disorder, remain within primary care or nonpsychiatric medical specialties. Psychiatric referral is often resented, unless accomplished early in the development of the disorder and with tactful collaboration between physician and psychiatrist. The degree of associated disability is very variable; some individuals dominate or manipulate family and social networks as a result of their symptoms, in contrast to a minority who function almost normally.

Diagnostic guidelines

For a definite diagnosis, both of the following should be present:

(a)   persistent belief in the presence of at least one serious physical illness underlying the presenting symptom or symptoms, even though repeated investigations and examinations have identified no adequate physical explanation, or a persistent preoccupation with a presumed deformity or disfigurement;

(b)   persistent refusal to accept the advice and reassurance of several different doctors that there is no physical illness or abnormality underlying the symptoms.

Includes: body dysmorphic disorder
         dysmorphophobia (nondelusional)
         hypochondriacal neurosis
         hypochondriasis
         nosophobia

Differential diagnosis
Differentiation from the following disorders is essential:

Somatization disorder
Emphasis is on the presence of the disorder itself and its future consequences, rather than on the individual symptoms as in somatization disorder. In hypochondriacal disorder, there is also likely to be preoccupation with only one or two possible physical disorders, which will be named consistently, rather than with the more numerous and often changing possibilities in somatization disorder. In hypochondriacal disorder there is no marked sex differential rate, nor are there any special familial connotations.

Depressive disorders
If depressive symptoms are particularly prominent and precede the development of hypochondriacal ideas, the depressive disorder may be primary.

Delusional disorders
The beliefs in hypochondriacal disorder do not have the same fixity as those in depressive and schizophrenic disorders accompanied by somatic delusions. A disorder in which the patient is convinced that he or she has an unpleasant appearance or is physically misshapen should be classified under delusional disorder (F22.–).

Anxiety and panic disorders
The somatic symptoms of anxiety are sometimes interpreted as signs of serious physical illness, but in these disorders the patients are usually reassured by physiological explanations, and convictions about the presence of physical illness do not develop.

One

F45.3   *Somatoform autonomic dysfunction*

The symptoms are presented by the patient as if they were due to a physical disorder of a system or organ that is largely or completely under autonomic innervation and control, i.e. the cardiovascular, gastrointestinal, or respiratory system. (Some aspects of the genitourinary system are also included here.) The most common and striking examples affect the cardiovascular system ('cardiac neurosis'), the respiratory system (psychogenic hyperventilation and hiccough) and the gastrointestinal system ('gastric neurosis' and 'nervous diarrhoea'). The symptoms are usually of two types, neither of which indicates a physical disorder of the organ or system concerned. The first type, upon which this diagnosis largely depends, is characterized by complaints based upon objective signs of autonomic arousal, such as palpitations, sweating, flushing, and tremor. The second type is characterized by more idiosyncratic, subjective, and nonspecific symptoms, such as sensations of fleeting aches and pains, burning, heaviness, tightness, and sensations of being bloated or distended; these are referred by the patient to a specific organ or system (as the autonomic symptoms may also be). It is the combination of clear autonomic involvement, additional nonspecific subjective complaints, and persistent referral to a particular organ or system as the cause of the disorder that gives the characteristic clinical picture.

In many patients with this disorder there will also be evidence of psychological stress, or current difficulties and problems that appear to be related to the disorder; however, this is not the case in a substantial proportion of patients who nevertheless clearly fulfil the criteria for this condition.

In some of these disorders, some minor disturbance of physiological function may also be present, such as hiccough, flatulence, and hyperventilation, but these do not of themselves disturb the essential physiological function of the relevant organ or system.

Diagnostic guidelines

Definite diagnosis requires all of the following:

(a)   symptoms of autonomic arousal, such as palpitations, sweating, tremor, flushing, which are persistent and troublesome;

(b)   additional subjective symptoms referred to a specific organ or system;

(c)   preoccupation with and distress about the possibility of a serious (but often unspecified) disorder of the stated organ or system, which does not respond to repeated explanation and reassurance by doctors;

(d)   no evidence of a significant disturbance of structure or function of the stated system or organ.

Differential diagnosis

Differentiation from generalized anxiety disorder is based on the predominance of the psychological, components of autonomic arousal, such as fear and anxious foreboding in generalized anxiety disorder, and the lack of a consistent physical focus for the other symptoms. In somatization disorders, autonomic symptoms may occur but they are neither prominent nor persistent in comparison with the many other sensations and feelings, and the symptoms are not so persistently attributed to one stated organ or system.

Excludes: psychological and behavioural factors associated with disorders or diseases classified elsewhere (F54)

A fifth character may be used to classify the individual disorders in this group, indicating the organ or system regarded by the patient as the origin of the symptoms:

F45.30 Heart and cardiovascular system
Includes: cardiac neurosis
             Da Costa's syndrome
             neurocirculatory asthenia

F45.31 Upper gastrointestinal tract
Includes: gastric neurosis
             psychogenic aerophagy, hiccough, dyspepsia, and pylorospasm

F45.32 Lower gastrointestinal tract
Includes: psychogenic flatulence, irritable bowel syndrome, and diarrhoea
             gas syndrome

F45.33 Respiratory system
Includes: psychogenic forms of cough and hyperventilation

F45.34 Genitourinary system
Includes: psychogenic increase of frequency of micturition and dysuria

F45.38 Other organ or system

One

F45.4 *Persistent somatoform pain disorder*

The predominant complaint is of persistent, severe, and distressing pain, which cannot be explained fully by a physiological process or a physical disorder. Pain occurs in association with emotional conflict or psychosocial problems that are sufficient to allow the conclusion that they are the main causative influences. The result is usually a marked increase in support and attention, either personal or medical.

Pain presumed to be of psychogenic origin occurring during the course of depressive disorder or schizophrenia should not be included here. Pain due to known or inferred psychophysiological mechanisms such as muscle tension pain or migraine, but still believed to have a psychogenic cause, should be coded by the use of F54 (psychological or behavioural factors associated with disorders or diseases classified elsewhere) plus an additional code from elsewhere in ICD-10 (e.g. migraine, G43.–).

Includes: psychalgia
psychogenic backache or headache
somatoform pain disorder

Differential diagnosis.

The commonest problem is to differentiate this disorder from the histrionic elaboration of organically caused pain. Patients with organic pain for whom a definite physical diagnosis has not yet been reached may easily become frightened or resentful, with resulting attention-seeking behaviour. A variety of aches and pains are common in somatization disorders but are not so persistent or so dominant over the other complaints.
Excludes: backache NOS (M54.9)
pain NOS (acute/chronic) (R52.–)
tension-type headache (G44.2)

F45.8 *Other somatoform disorders*

In these disorders the presenting complaints are not mediated through the autonomic nervous system, and are limited to specific systems or parts of the body. This is in contrast to the multiple and often changing complaints of the origin of symptoms and distress found in somatization disorder (F45.0) and undifferentiated somatoform disorder (F45.1). Tissue damage is not involved.

Any other disorders of sensation not due to physical disorders, which are closely associated in time with stressful events or problems, or which result in significantly increased attention for the patient, either personal or medical, should also be classified here. Sensations of swelling, movements on the skin, and paræsthesias (tingling and/or numbness) are common examples. Disorders such as the following should also be included here:

(a) 'globus hystericus' (a feeling of a lump in the throat causing dysphagia) and other forms of dysphagia;

(b) psychogenic torticollis, and other disorders of spasmodic movements (but excluding Tourette's syndrome);

(c) psychogenic pruritus (but excluding specific skin lesions such as alopecia, dermatitis, eczema, or urticaria of psychogenic origin (F54));

(d) psychogenic dysmenorrhoea (but excluding dyspareunia (F52.6) and frigidity (F52.0));

(e) teeth-grinding

F45.9　Somatoform disorder, unspecified
Includes: unspecified psychophysiological or psychosomatic disorder

F48　Other neurotic disorders

F48.0　Neurasthenia
Considerable cultural variations occur in the presentation of this disorder; two main types occur, with substantial overlap. In one type, the main feature is a complaint of increased fatigue after mental effort, often associated with some decrease in occupational performance or coping efficiency in daily tasks. The mental fatiguability is typically described as an unpleasant intrusion of distracting associations or recollections, difficulty in concentrating, and generally inefficient thinking. In the other type, the emphasis is on feelings of bodily or physical weakness and exhaustion after only minimal effort, accompanied by a feeling of muscular aches and pains and inability to relax. In both types, a variety of other unpleasant physical feelings, such as dizziness, tension headaches, and a sense of general instability, is common. Worry about decreasing mental and bodily well-being, irritability, anhedonia, and varying minor degrees of both depression and anxiety are all common. Sleep is often disturbed in its initial and middle phases but hypersomnia may also be prominent.

Diagnostic guidelines
Definite diagnosis requires the following:

(a) either persistent and distressing complaints of increased fatigue after mental effort, or persistent and distressing complaints of bodily weakness and exhaustion after minimal effort;

(b)   at least two of the following:
- feelings of muscular aches and pains
- dizziness
- tension headaches
- sleep disturbance
- inability to relax
- irritability
- dyspepsia;

(c)   any autonomic or depressive symptoms present are not sufficiently persistent and severe to fulfil the criteria for any of the more specific disorders in this classification.

Includes: fatigue syndrome

Differential diagnosis

In many countries neurasthenia is not generally used as a diagnostic category. Many of the cases so diagnosed in the past would meet the current
criteria for depressive disorder or anxiety disorder. There are, however,
cases that fit the description of neurasthenia better than that of any other
neurotic syndrome, and such cases seem to be more frequent in some
cultures than in others. If the diagnostic category of neurasthenia is used,
an attempt should be made first to rule out a depressive illness or an anxiety disorder. Hallmarks of the syndrome are the patient's emphasis on
fatiguability and weakness and concern about lowered mental and physical efficiency (in contrast to the somatoform disorders, where bodily
complaints and preoccupation with physical disease dominate the picture). If the neurasthenic syndrome develops in the aftermath of a physical illness (particularly influenza, viral hepatitis, or infectious mononu-
cleosis), the diagnosis of the latter should also be recorded.

Excludes: asthenia NOS (R53)
burn-out (Z73.0)
malaise and fatigue (R53)
postviral fatigue syndrome (G93.3)
psychasthenia (F48.8)

F48.1   *Depersonalization–derealization syndrome*

A disorder in which the sufferer complains that his or her mental activity, body, and/or surroundings are changed in their quality, so as to be
unreal, remote, or automatized. Individuals may feel that they are no
longer doing their own thinking, imaging, or remembering; that their

movements and behaviour are somehow not their own; that their body seems lifeless, detached, or otherwise anomalous; and that their surroundings seem to lack colour and life and appear as artificial, or as a stage on which people are acting contrived roles. In some cases, they may feel as if they were viewing themselves from a distance or as if they were dead. The complaint of loss of emotions is the most frequent among these varied phenomena.

The number of individuals who experience this disorder in a pure or isolated form is small. More commonly, depersonalization–derealization phenomena occur in the context of depressive illnesses, phobic disorder, and obsessive-compulsive disorder. Elements of the syndrome may also occur in mentally healthy individuals in states of fatigue, sensory deprivation, hallucinogen intoxication, or as a hypnogogic/ hypnopompic phenomenon. The depersonalization–derealization phenomena are similar to the so-called 'near-death experiences' associated with moments of extreme danger to life.

Diagnostic guidelines

For a definite diagnosis, there must be either or both of (a) and (b), plus (c) and (d):

(a)   depersonalization symptoms, i.e. the individual feels that his or her own feelings and/or experiences are detached, distant, not his or her own, lost, etc;

(b)   derealization symptoms, i.e. objects, people, and/or surroundings seem unreal, distant, artificial, colourless, lifeless, etc;

(c)   an acceptance that this is a subjective and spontaneous change, not imposed by outside forces or other people (i.e. insight);

(d)   a clear sensorium and absence of toxic confusional state or epilepsy.

Differential diagnosis

The disorder must be differentiated from other disorders in which 'change of personality' is experienced or presented, such as schizophrenia (delusions of transformation or passivity and control experiences), dissociative disorders (where awareness of change is lacking), and some instances of early dementia. The preictal aura of temporal lobe epilepsy and some postictal states may include depersonalization and derealization syndromes as secondary phenomena.

If the depersonalization-derealization syndrome occurs as part of a diagnosable depressive, phobic, obsessive-compulsive, or schizophrenic disorder, the latter should be given precedence as the main diagnosis.

F48.8 *Other specified neurotic disorders*

This category includes mixed disorders of behaviour, beliefs, and emotions which are of uncertain etiology and nosological status and that occur with particular frequency in certain cultures; examples include Dhat syndrome (undue concern about the debilitating effects of the passage of semen), koro (anxiety and fear that the penis will retract into the abdomen and cause death), and latah (imitative and automatic response behaviour). The strong association of these syndromes with locally accepted cultural beliefs and patterns of behaviour indicates that they are probably best regarded as not delusional.

Includes: Briquet's disorder
Dhat syndrome
koro
latah
occupational neurosis, including writer's cramp
psychasthenia
psychasthenic neurosis
psychogenic syncope

F48.9 *Neurotic disorder, unspecified*
Includes: neurosis NOS

F50–F59   Behavioural syndromes associated with physiological disturbances and physical factors

F50   Eating disorders
    F50.0   Anorexia nervosa
    F50.1   Atypical anorexia nervosa
    F50.2   Bulimia nervosa
    F50.3   Atypical bulimia nervosa
    F50.4   Overeating associated with other psychological disturbances
    F50.5   Vomiting associated with other psychological disturbances
    F50.8   Other eating disorders
    F50.9   Eating disorder, unspecified

F51   Nonorganic sleep disorders
    F51.0   Nonorganic insomnia
    F51.1   Nonorganic hypersomnia
    F51.2   Nonorganic disorder of the sleep–wake schedule
    F51.3   Sleepwalking [somnambulism]
    F51.4   Sleep terrors [night terrors]
    F51.5   Nightmares
    F51.8   Other nonorganic sleep disorders
    F51.9   Nonorganic sleep disorder, unspecified

F52   Sexual dysfunction, not caused by organic disorder or disease
    F52.0   Lack or loss of sexual desire
    F52.1   Sexual aversion and lack of sexual enjoyment
      .10   Sexual aversion
      .11   Lack of sexual enjoyment
    F52.2   Failure of genital response
    F52.3   Orgasmic dysfunction
    F52.4   Premature ejaculation
    F52.5   Nonorganic vaginismus
    F52.6   Nonorganic dyspareunia
    F52.7   Excessive sexual drive
    F52.8   Other sexual dysfunction, not caused by organic disorder or disease
    F52.9   Unspecified sexual dysfunction, not caused by organic disorder or disease

F53   Mental and behavioural disorders associated with the puerperium, not elsewhere classified

One

F53.0 Mild mental and behavioural disorders associated with the puerperium, not elsewhere classified

F53.1 Severe mental and behavioural disorders associated with the puerperium, not elsewhere classified

F53.8 Other mental and behavioural disorders associated with the puerperium, not elsewhere classified

F53.9 Puerperal mental disorder, unspecified

F54 Psychological and behavioural factors associated with disorders or diseases classified elsewhere

F55 Abuse of non-dependence-producing substances

F55.0 Antidepressants

F55.1 Laxatives

F55.2 Analgesics

F55.3 Antacids

F55.4 Vitamins

F55.5 Steroids or hormones

F55.6 Specific herbal or folk remedies

F55.8 Other substances that do not produce dependence

F55.9 Unspecified

F59 Unspecified behavioural syndromes associated with physiological disturbances and physical factors

F50   Eating disorders

Under the heading of eating disorders, two important and clear-cut syndromes are described: anorexia nervosa and bulimia nervosa. Less specific bulimic disorders also deserve a place, as does overeating when it is associated with psychological disturbances. A brief note is provided on vomiting associated with psychological disturbances.

Excludes: anorexia or loss of appetite NOS (R63.0)
feeding difficulties and mismanagement (R63.3)
feeding disorder of infancy and childhood (F98.2)
pica in children (F98.3)

F50.0   Anorexia nervosa

Anorexia nervosa is a disorder characterized by deliberate weight loss, induced and/or sustained by the patient. The disorder occurs most commonly in adolescent girls and young women, but adolescent boys and young men may be affected more rarely, as may children approaching puberty and older women up to the menopause. Anorexia nervosa constitutes an independent syndrome in the following sense:

(a)   the clinical features of the syndrome are easily recognized, so that diagnosis is reliable with a high level of agreement between clinicians;

(b)   follow-up studies have shown that, among patients who do not recover, a considerable number continue to show the same main features of anorexia nervosa, in a chronic form.

Although the fundamental causes of anorexia nervosa remain elusive, there is growing evidence that interacting sociocultural and biological factors contribute to its causation, as do less specific psychological mechanisms and a vulnerability of personality. The disorder is associated with undernutrition of varying severity, with resulting secondary endocrine and metabolic changes and disturbances of bodily function. There remains some doubt as to whether the characteristic endocrine disorder is entirely due to the undernutrition and the direct effect of various behaviours that have brought it about (e.g. restricted dietary choice, excessive exercise and alterations in body composition, induced vomiting and purgation and the consequent electrolyte disturbances), or whether uncertain factors are also involved.

Diagnostic guidelines
For a definite diagnosis, all the following are required:

(a)   Body weight is maintained at least 15% below that expected (either lost or never achieved), or Quetelet's body-mass index[1] is 17.5 or less. Prepubertal patients may show failure to make the expected weight gain during the period of growth.

(b)   The weight loss is self-induced by avoidance of 'fattening foods'. One or more of the following may also be present: self-induced vomiting; self-induced purging; excessive exercise; use of appetite suppressants and/or diuretics.

(c)   There is body-image distortion in the form of a specific psychopathology whereby a dread of fatness persists as an intrusive, overvalued idea and the patient imposes a low weight threshold on himself or herself.

(d)   A widespread endocrine disorder involving the hypothalamic–pituitary–gonadal axis is manifest in women as amenorrhoea and in men as a loss of sexual interest and potency. (An apparent exception is the persis-

[1]   Quetelet's body-mass index $= \dfrac{\text{weight (kg)}}{[\text{height (m)}]^2}$ to be used for age 16 or more.

tence of vaginal bleeds in anorexic women who are receiving replacement hormonal therapy, most commonly taken as a contraceptive pill.) There may also be elevated levels of growth hormone, raised levels of cortisol, changes in the peripheral metabolism of the thyroid hormone, and abnormalities of insulin secretion.

(e) If onset is prepubertal, the sequence of pubertal events is delayed or even arrested (growth ceases; in girls the breasts do not develop and there is a primary amenorrhoea; in boys the genitals remain juvenile). With recovery, puberty is often completed normally, but the menarche is late.

Differential diagnosis

There may be associated depressive or obsessional symptoms, as well as features of a personality disorder, which may make differentiation difficult and/or require the use of more than one diagnostic code. Somatic causes of weight loss in young patients that must be distinguished include chronic debilitating diseases, brain tumors, and intestinal disorders such as Crohn's disease or a malabsorption syndrome.

Excludes: loss of appetite (R63.0)
psychogenic loss of appetite (F50.8)

F50.1 Atypical anorexia nervosa

This term should be used for those individuals in whom one or more of the key features of anorexia nervosa (F50.0), such as amenorrhoea or significant weight loss, is absent, but who otherwise present a fairly typical clinical picture. Such people are usually encountered in psychiatric liaison services in general hospitals or in primary care. Patients who have all the key symptoms but to only a mild degree may also be best described by this term. This term should not be used for eating disorders that resemble anorexia nervosa but that are due to known physical illness.

F50.2 Bulimia nervosa

Bulimia nervosa is a syndrome characterized by repeated bouts of overeating and an excessive preoccupation with the control of body weight, leading the patient to adopt extreme measures so as to mitigate the 'fattening' effects of ingested food. The term should be restricted to the form of the disorder that is related to anorexia nervosa by virtue of sharing the same psychopathology. The age and sex distribution is similar to that of anorexia nervosa, but the age of presentation tends to be slightly later. The disorder may be viewed as a sequel to persistent anorexia nervosa (although the reverse sequence may also occur). A previously anorexic patient may first appear to improve as a result of weight gain and possibly a return of menstruation, but a pernicious pattern of overeating and vomiting then becomes established. Repeated vomiting is likely to give rise to disturbances of body electrolytes, physical complications (tetany, epileptic seizures, cardiac arrhythmias, muscular weakness), and further severe loss of weight.

Diagnostic guidelines

For a definite diagnosis, all the following are required:

(a) There is a persistent preoccupation with eating, and an irresistible craving for food; the patient succumbs to episodes of overeating in which large amounts of food are consumed in short periods of time.

(b) The patient attempts to counteract the 'fattening' effects of food by one or more of the following: self-induced vomiting; purgative abuse, alternating periods of starvation; use of drugs such as appetite suppressants, thyroid preparations or diuretics. When bulimia occurs in diabetic patients they may choose to neglect their insulin treatment.

(c) The psychopathology consists of a morbid dread of fatness and the patient sets herself or himself a sharply defined weight threshold, well below the premorbid weight that constitutes the optimum or healthy weight in the opinion of the physician. There is often, but not always, a history of an earlier episode of anorexia nervosa, the interval between the two disorders ranging from a few months to several years. This earlier episode may have been fully expressed, or may have assumed a minor cryptic form with a moderate loss of weight and/or a transient phase of amenorrhoea.

Includes: bulimia NOS
         hyperorexia nervosa

Differential diagnosis

Bulimia nervosa must be differentiated from:

(a) upper gastrointestinal disorders leading to repeated vomiting (the characteristic psychopathology is absent);

(b) a more general abnormality of personality (the eating disorder may coexist with alcohol dependence and petty offenses such as shoplifting);

(c) depressive disorder (bulimic patients often experience depressive symptoms).

F50.3   Atypical bulimia nervosa

This term should be used for those individuals in whom one or more of the key features listed for bulimia nervosa (F50.2) is absent, but who otherwise present a fairly typical clinical picture. Most commonly this applies to people with normal or even excessive weight but with typical periods of overeating followed by vomiting or purging. Partial syndromes together with depressive symptoms are also not uncommon, but if the depressive symptoms justify a separate diagnosis of a depressive disorder two separate diagnoses should be made.

Includes: normal weight bulimia

F50.4   Overeating associated with other psychological disturbances

Overeating that has led to obesity as a reaction to distressing events should be coded here. Bereavements, accidents, surgical operations, and emotionally distressing events may be followed by a 'reactive obesity', especially in individuals predisposed to weight gain.

Obesity as a cause of psychological disturbance should not be coded here. Obesity may cause the individual to feel sensitive about his or her appearance and give rise to a lack of confidence in personal relationships; the subjective appraisal of body size may be exaggerated. Obesity as a cause of psychological disturbance should be coded in a category such as F38.– (other mood [affective] disorders), F41.2 (mixed anxiety and depressive disorder), or F48.9 (neurotic disorder, unspecified), plus a code from E66.– of ICD-10 within Axis Four, to indicate the type of obesity.

Obesity as an undesirable effect of long-term treatment with neuroleptic antidepressants or other type of medication should not be coded here, but in Axis Four under E66.1 (drug-induced obesity) plus an additional code from Chapter XX (External causes) of ICD-10, to identify the drug.

Obesity may be the motivation for dieting, which in turn results in minor affective symptoms (anxiety, restlessness, weakness, and irritability) or, more rarely, severe depressive symptoms ('dieting depression'). The appropriate code from F30–F39 or F40–F49 should be used to cover the symptoms as above, plus F50.8 (other eating disorder) to indicate the dieting, plus a code from E66.– in Axis Four to indicate the type of obesity.

Includes: psychogenic overeating
Excludes: obesity (E66.–)
                   polyphagia NOS (R63.2)

F50.5   *Vomiting associated with other psychological disturbances*

Apart from the self-induced vomiting of bulimia nervosa, repeated vomiting may occur in dissociative disorders (F44.–), in hypochondriacal disorder (F45.2) when vomiting may be one of several bodily symptoms, and in pregnancy when emotional factors may contribute to recurrent nausea and vomiting.

Includes: psychogenic hyperemesis gravidarum
                 psychogenic vomiting
Excludes: nausea and vomiting NOS (R11)

F50.8   *Other eating disorders*

Includes: pica of nonorganic origin in adults
                 psychogenic loss of appetite
Excludes: feeding disorders (often in young children) that fail to meet criteria for any specified eating disorder (F99.2)

F50.9   *Eating disorder, unspecified*

F51   **Nonorganic sleep disorders**

This group of disorders includes:

(a)   dyssomnias: primarily psychogenic conditions in which the predominant disturbance is in the amount, quality, or timing of sleep due to emotional causes, i.e. insomnia, hypersomnia, and disorder of sleep-wake schedule; and

(b)   parasomnias: abnormal episodic events occurring during sleep; in childhood these are related mainly to the child's development, while in adulthood they are predominantly psychogenic, i.e. sleepwalking, sleep terrors, and nightmares.

This section includes only those sleep disorders in which emotional causes are considered to be a primary factor. Sleep disorders of organic origin are coded in Axis Four such as Kleine–Levin syndrome (G47.8) are coded in Chapter VI (G47.–) of ICD-10. Nonpsychogenic disorders including narcolepsy and cataplexy (G47.4) and disorders of the sleep–wake schedule (G47.2) are also listed in Chapter VI and will be coded in Axis Four, as are sleep apnoea (G47.3) and episodic movement disorders that include nocturnal myoclonus (G25.3). Finally, enuresis (F98.0) is listed with other emotional and behavioural disorders with onset specific to childhood and adolescence that are coded in Axis One, while primary nocturnal enuresis (R33.8), which is considered to be due to a maturational delay of bladder control during sleep, is listed in Chapter XVIII of ICD-10 among the symptoms involving the urinary system, and coded in Axis Four.

In many cases, a disturbance of sleep is one of the symptoms of another disorder, either mental or physical. Even when a specific sleep disorder appears to be clinically independent, a number of associated psychiatric and/or physical factors may contribute to its occurrence. Whether a sleep disorder in a given individual is an independent condition or simply one of the features of another disorder (classified elsewhere in Chapter V or in other chapters of ICD–10 should be determined on the basis of its clinical presentation and course, as well as of therapeutic considerations and priorities at the time of the consultation. In any event, whenever the disturbance of sleep is among the predominant complaints, a sleep disorder should be diagnosed. Generally, however, it is preferable to list the diagnosis of the specific sleep disorder along with as many other pertinent diagnoses as are necessary to describe adequately the psychopathology and/or pathophysiology involved in a given case.

Excludes: sleep disorders (organic) (G47.–)

F51.0   *Nonorganic insomnia*

Insomnia is a condition of unsatisfactory quantity and/or quality of sleep, which persists for a considerable period of time. The actual degree of deviation from what is generally considered as a normal amount of sleep should not be the primary consideration in the diagnosis of insomnia, because some individuals (the so-called short sleepers) obtain a minimal amount of sleep and yet do not consider themselves as insomniacs. Conversely, there are people who suffer immensely from the poor quality of their sleep, while sleep quantity is judged subjectively and/or objectively as within normal limits.

Among insomniacs, difficulty falling asleep is the most prevalent complaint, followed by difficulty staying asleep and early final wakening. Usually, however, patients report a combination of these complaints. Typically, insomnia develops at a time of increased life-stress. When insomnia is repeatedly experienced, it can lead to an increased fear of sleeplessness and a preoccupation with its consequences. This creates a vicious circle which tends to perpetuate the individual's problem.

Individuals with insomnia describe themselves as feeling tense, anxious, worried, or depressed at bedtime, and as though their thoughts are racing. They frequently ruminate over getting enough sleep, personal problems, health status, and even death. Often they attempt to cope with their tension by taking medication or alcohol. In the morning, they frequently report feeling physically and mentally tired; during the day, they characteristically feel depressed, worried, tense, irritable, and preoccupied with themselves.

Children are often said to have difficulty sleeping when in reality the problem is a difficulty in the management of bedtime routines (rather than of sleep *per se*); such bedtime difficulties should not be coded here. Rather they should be coded under F99.1 or F99.2. If part of a broader picture of inadequate parental supervision and control they should also be coded under 4.1 in Axis Five.

Diagnostic guidelines
The following are essential clinical features for a definite diagnosis:

(a) the complaint is either of difficulty falling asleep or maintaining sleep, or of poor quality of sleep;

(b) the sleep disturbance has occurred at least three times per week for at least 1 month;

(c) there is preoccupation with the sleeplessness and excessive concern over its consequences at night and during the day;

(d) the unsatisfactory quantity and/or quality of sleep either causes marked distress or interferes with ordinary activities in daily living.

Whenever unsatisfactory quantity and/or quality of sleep is the patient's only complaint, the disorder should be coded here. The presence of other psychiatric symptoms such as depression, anxiety or obsessions does not invalidate the diagnosis of insomnia, provided that insomnia is the primary complaint or the chronicity and severity of insomnia cause the patient to perceive it as the primary disorder. Other coexisting disorders should be coded if they are sufficiently marked and persistent to justify treatment in their own right. It should be noted that most chronic insomniacs are usually preoccupied with their sleep disturbance and deny the existence of any emotional problems. Thus, careful clinical assessment is necessary before ruling out a psychological basis for the complaint.

Insomnia is a common symptom of other mental disorders, such as affective, neurotic, organic, and eating disorders, substance use, and schizophrenia, and of other sleep disorders such as nightmares. Insomnia may also be associated with physical disorders in which there is pain and discomfort or with taking certain medications. If insomnia occurs only as one of the multiple symptoms of a mental disorder or a physical condition, i.e. does not dominate the clinical picture, the diagnosis should be limited to that of the underlying mental or physical disorder. Moreover, the diagnosis of another sleep disorder, such as nightmare, disorder of the sleep–wake schedule, sleep apnoea and nocturnal myoclonus, should be made only when these disorders lead to a reduction in the quantity or quality of sleep. However, in all of the above instances, if insomnia is one of the major complaints and is perceived as a condition in itself, the present code should be added after that of the principal diagnosis.

The present code does not apply to so-called 'transient insomnia'. Transient disturbances of sleep are a normal part of everyday life. Thus, a few nights of sleeplessness related to a psychosocial stressor would not be coded here, but could be considered as part of an acute stress reaction (F43.0) or adjustment disorder (F43.2) if accompanied by other clinically significant features.

F51.1   Nonorganic hypersomnia

Hypersomnia is defined as a condition of either excessive daytime sleepiness and sleep attacks (not accounted for by an inadequate amount of sleep) or prolonged transition to the fully aroused state upon awakening. When no definite evidence of organic etiology can be found, this condition is usually associated with mental disorders. It is often found to be a symptom of a bipolar affective disorder currently depressed (F31.3, F31.4 or F31.5), a recurrent depressive disorder (F33.–) or a depressive episode (F32.–). At times, however, the criteria for the diagnosis of another mental disorder cannot be met, although there is often some evidence of a psychopathological basis for the complaint.

Some patients will themselves make the connection between their tendency to fall asleep at inappropriate times and certain unpleasant daytime experiences. Others will deny such a connection even when a skilled clinician identifies the presence of these experiences. In other cases, no emotional or other psychological factors can be readily identified, but the presumed absence of organic factors suggests that the hypersomnia is most likely of psychogenic origin.

Diagnostic guidelines

The following clinical features are essential for a definite diagnosis:

(a)   excessive daytime sleepiness or sleep attacks, not accounted for by an inadequate amount of sleep, and/or prolonged transition to the fully aroused state upon awakening (sleep drunkenness);

(b) sleep disturbance occurring daily for more than 1 month or for recurrent periods of shorter duration, causing either marked distress or interference with ordinary activities in daily living;

(c) absence of auxiliary symptoms of narcolepsy (cataplexy, sleep paralysis, hypnagogic hallucinations) or of clinical evidence for sleep apnoea (nocturnal breath cessation, typical intermittent snorting sounds, etc.);

(d) absence of any neurological or medical condition of which daytime somnolence may be symptomatic.

If hypersomnia occurs only as one of the symptoms of a mental disorder, such as an affective disorder, the diagnosis should be that of the underlying disorder. The diagnosis of psychogenic hypersomnia should be added, however, if hypersomnia is the predominant complaint in patients with other mental disorders. When another diagnosis cannot be made, the present code should be used alone.

Differential diagnosis
Differentiating hypersomnia from narcolepsy is essential. In narcolepsy (G47.4), one or more auxiliary symptoms such as cataplexy, sleep paralysis, and hypnagogic hallucinations are usually present; the sleep attacks are irresistible and more refreshing; and nocturnal sleep is fragmented and curtailed. By contrast, daytime sleep attacks in hypersomnia are usually fewer per day, although each of longer duration; the patient is often able to prevent their occurrence; nocturnal sleep is usually prolonged, and there is a marked difficulty in achieving the fully aroused state upon awakening (sleep drunkenness).

It is important to differentiate nonorganic hypersomnia from hypersomnia related to sleep apnoea and other organic hypersomnias. In addition to the symptom of excessive daytime sleepiness, most patients with sleep apnoea have a history of nocturnal cessation of breathing, typical intermittent snorting sounds, obesity, hypertension, impotence, cognitive impairment, nocturnal hypermotility and profuse sweating, morning headaches and incoordination. When there is a strong suspicion of sleep apnoea, confirmation of the diagnosis and quantification of the apnoeic events by means of sleep laboratory recordings should be considered.

Hypersomnia due to a definable organic cause (encephalitis, meningitis, concussion and other brain damage, brain tumours, cerebrovascular lesions, degenerative and other neurologic diseases, metabolic disorders, toxic conditions, endocrine abnormalities, post-radiation syndrome) can be differentiated from nonorganic hypersomnia by the presence of the insulting organic factor, as evidenced by the patient's clinical presentation and the results of appropriate laboratory tests.

F51.2   *Nonorganic disorder of the sleep–wake schedule*

A disorder of the sleep–wake schedule is defined as a lack of synchrony between the individual's sleep–wake schedule and the desired sleep–wake schedule for the environment, resulting in a complaint of either insomnia or hypersomnia. This disorder may be either psychogenic or of presumed organic origin, depending on the relative contribution of psychological or organic factors. Individuals with disorganized and variable sleeping and waking times most often present with significant psychological disturbance, usually in association with various psychiatric conditions such as personality disorders and affective disorders. In individuals who frequently change work shifts or travel across time zones, the circadian dysregulation is basically biological, although a strong emotional component may also be operating since many such individuals are distressed. Finally, in some individuals there is a phase advance to the desired sleep–wake schedule, which may be due to either an intrinsic malfunction of the circadian oscillator (biological clock) or an abnormal processing of the time-cues that drive the biological clock (the latter may in fact be related to an emotional and/or cognitive disturbance).

The present code is reserved for those disorders of the sleep–wake schedule in which psychological factors play the most important role, whereas cases of presumed organic origin should be classified under G47.2 in Axis Four, i.e. as non-psychogenic disorders of the sleep–wake schedule. Whether or not psychological factors are of primary importance and, therefore, whether the present code or G47.2 should be used is a matter for clinical judgement in each case.

Diagnostic guidelines

The following clinical features are essential for a definite diagnosis:

(a)   the individual's sleep–wake pattern is out of synchrony with the sleep–wake schedule that is normal for a particular society and shared by most people in the same cultural environment;

(b)   insomnia during the major sleep period and hypersomnia during the waking period are experienced nearly every day for at least 1 month or recurrently for shorter periods of time;

(c)   the unsatisfactory quantity, quality, and timing of sleep cause marked distress or interfere with ordinary activities in daily living.

Whenever there is no identifiable psychiatric or physical cause of the disorder, the present code should be used alone. None the less, the presence of psychiatric symptoms such as anxiety, depression, or hypomania does not invalidate the diagnosis of a nonorganic disorder of the sleep–wake schedule, provided that this disorder is predominant in the patient's clinical picture. When other psychiatric symptoms are sufficiently marked and persistent, the specific mental disorder(s) should be diagnosed separately.

Includes: psychogenic inversion of circadian, nyctohemeral, or sleep rhythm

F51.3   *Sleepwalking [somnambulism]*

Sleepwalking or somnambulism is a state of altered consciousness in which phenomena of sleep and wakefulness are combined. During a sleepwalking episode the individual arises from bed, usually during the first third of nocturnal sleep, and walks about, exhibiting low levels of awareness, reactivity, and motor skill. A sleepwalker will sometimes leave the bedroom and at times may actually walk out of the house, and is thus exposed to considerable risks of injury during the episode. Most often, however, he or she will return quietly to bed, either unaided or when gently led by another person. Upon awakening either from the sleepwalking episode or the next morning, there is usually no recall of the event.

Sleepwalking and sleep terrors (F51.4) are very closely related. Both are considered as disorders of arousal, particularly arousal from the deepest stages of sleep (stages 3 and 4). Many individuals have a positive family history for either condition as well as a personal history of having experienced both. Moreover, both conditions are much more common in childhood, which indicates the role of developmental factors in their etiology. In addition, in some cases, the onset of these conditions coincides with a febrile illness. When they continue beyond childhood or are first observed in adulthood, both conditions tend to be associated with significant psychological disturbance. Based upon the clinical and pathogenetic similarities between sleepwalking and sleep terrors, and the fact that the differential diagnosis of these disorders is usually a matter of which of the two is predominant, they have both been considered recently to be part of the same nosologic continuum. For consistency with tradition, however, as well as to emphasize the differences in the intensity of clinical manifestations, separate codes are provided in this classification.

Diagnostic guidelines
The following clinical features are essential for a definite diagnosis:

(a)   the predominant symptom is one or more episodes of rising from bed, usually during the first third of nocturnal sleep, and walking about;

(b)   during an episode, the individual has a blank, staring face, is relatively unresponsive to the efforts of others to influence the event or to communicate with him or her, and can be awakened only with considerable difficulty;

(c)   upon awakening (either from an episode or the next morning), the individual has no recollection of the episode;

(d)   within several minutes of awakening from the episode, there is no impairment of mental activity or behaviour, although there may initially be a short period of some confusion and disorientation;

(e)   there is no evidence of an organic mental disorder such as dementia, or a physical disorder such as epilepsy.

Differential diagnosis
Sleepwalking should be differentiated from psychomotor epileptic seizures. Psychomotor epilepsy very seldom occurs only at night. During the epileptic attack the individual is completely unresponsive to environmental stimuli, and perseverative movements such as swallowing and rubbing the hands are common. The presence of epileptic discharges in the EEG confirms the diagnosis, although a seizure disorder does not preclude coexisting sleepwalking.

Dissociative fugue (see F44.1) must also be differentiated from sleepwalking. In dissociative disorders the episodes are much longer in duration and patients are more alert and capable of complex and purposeful behaviours. Further, these disorders are rare in children and typically begin during the hours of wakefulness.

F51.4   Sleep terrors [night terrors]
Sleep terrors or night terrors are nocturnal episodes of extreme terror and panic associated with intense vocalization, motility, and high levels of autonomic discharge. The individual sits up or gets up with a panicky scream, usually during the first third of nocturnal sleep, often rushing to the door as if trying to escape, although he or she very seldom leaves the room. Efforts of others to influence the sleep terror event may actually lead to more intense fear, since the individual not only is relatively unresponsive to such efforts but may become disoriented for a few minutes. Upon awaking there is usually no recollection of the episode. Because of

these clinical characteristics, individuals are at great risk of injury during the episodes of sleep terrors.

Sleep terrors and sleepwalking (F51.3) are closely related: genetic, developmental, organic, and psychological factors all play a role in their development, and the two conditions share the same clinical and patho-physiological characteristics. On the basis of their many similarities, these two conditions have been considered recently to be part of the same nosologic continuum.

Diagnostic guidelines
The following clinical features are essential for a definite diagnosis:

(a) the predominant symptom is that one or more episodes of awakening from sleep begin with a panicky scream, and are characterized by intense anxiety, body motility, and autonomic hyperactivity, such as tachycardia, rapid breathing, dilated pupils, and sweating;

(b) these repeated episodes typically last 1–10 minutes and usually occur during the first third of nocturnal sleep;

(c) there is relative unresponsiveness to efforts of others to influence the sleep terror event and such efforts are almost invariably followed by at least several minutes of disorientation and perseverative movements;

(d) recall of the event, if any, is minimal (usually limited to one or two frag-mentary mental images);

(e) there is no evidence of a physical disorder, such as brain tumour or epilepsy.

Differential diagnosis
Sleep terrors should be differentiated from nightmares. The latter are the common 'bad dreams' with limited, if any, vocalization and body motili-ty. In contrast to sleep terrors, nightmares occur at any time of the night, and the individual is quite easy to arouse and has a very detailed and vivid recall of the event.

In differentiating sleep terrors from epileptic seizures, the physician should keep in mind that seizures very seldom occur only during the night; an abnormal clinical EEG, however, favours the diagnosis of epilepsy.

F51.5   Nightmares
Nightmares are dream experiences loaded with anxiety or fear, of which the individual has very detailed recall. The dream experiences are extremely vivid and usually include themes involving threats to survival,

security, or self-esteem. Quite often there is a recurrence of the same or similar frightening nightmare themes. During a typical episode there is a degree of autonomic discharge but no appreciable vocalization or body motility. Upon awakening, the individual rapidly becomes alert and oriented. He or she can fully communicate with others, usually giving a detailed account of the dream experience both immediately and the next morning.

In children, there is no consistently associated psychological disturbance, as childhood nightmares are usually related to a specific phase of emotional development. In contrast, adults with nightmares are often found to have significant psychological disturbance, usually in the form of a personality disorder. The use of certain psychotropic drugs such as reserpine, thioridazine, tricyclic antidepressants, and benzodiazepines has also been found to contribute to the occurrence of nightmares. Moreover, abrupt withdrawal of drugs such as non-benzodiazepine hypnotics, which suppress REM sleep (the stage of sleep related to dreaming), may lead to enhanced dreaming and nightmare through REM rebound.

Diagnostic guidelines
The following clinical features are essential for a definite diagnosis:

(a)   awakening from nocturnal sleep or naps with detailed and vivid recall of intensely frightening dreams, usually involving threats to survival, security, or self-esteem; the awakening may occur at any time during the sleep period, but typically during the second half;

(b)   upon awakening from the frightening dreams, the individual rapidly becomes oriented and alert;

(c)   the dream experience itself, and the resulting disturbance of sleep, cause marked distress to the individual.

Includes: dream anxiety disorder

Differential diagnosis
It is important to differentiate nightmares from sleep terrors. In the latter, the episodes occur during the first third of the sleep period and are marked by intense anxiety, panicky screams, excessive body motility, and extreme autonomic discharge. Further, in sleep terrors there is no detailed recollection of the dream, either immediately following the episode or upon awakening in the morning.

F51.8   *Other nonorganic sleep disorders*

F51.9   *Nonorganic sleep disorder, unspecified*
          Includes: emotional sleep disorder NOS

F52   Sexual dysfunction, not caused by organic disorder or disease

F52.0   *Lack or loss of sexual desire*

F52.1   *Sexual aversion and lack of sexual enjoyment*

F52.2   *Failure of genital response*

F52.3   *Orgasmic dysfunction*

F52.4   *Premature ejaculation*

F52.5   *Nonorganic vaginismus*

F52.6   *Nonorganic dyspareunia*

F52.7   *Excessive sexual drive*

F52.8   *Other sexual dysfunction, not caused by organic disorder or disease*

F52.9   *Unspecified sexual dysfunction, not caused by organic disorder or disease*

F53   Mental and behavioural disorders associated with the puerperium, not elsewhere classified

F53.0   *Mild mental and behavioural disorders associated with the puerperium, not elsewhere classified*

F53.1   *Severe mental and behavioural disorders associated with the puerperium, not elsewhere classified*

F53.8   *Other mental and behavioural disorders associated with the puerperium, not elsewhere classified*

F53.9   Puerperal mental disorder, unspecified

F54   Psychological and behavioural factors associated with disorders or diseases classified elsewhere

This category should be used to record the presence of psychological or behavioural influences thought to have played a major part in the manifestation of physical disorders that can be classified in Axis Four by using diagnoses from other chapters of ICD-10. Any resulting mental disturbances are usually mild and often prolonged (such as worry, emotional conflict, apprehension), and do not of themselves justify the use of any of the categories described in the rest of this book. An additional code should be used to identify the physical disorder. (In the rare instances in which an overt psychiatric disorder is thought to have caused a physical disorder, a second additional code should be used to record the psychiatric disorder.)

Examples of the use of this category are: asthma (F54 plus J45.–); dermatitis and eczema (F54 plus L23–L25); gastric ulcer (F54 plus K25.–); mucous colitis (F54 plus K58.–); ulcerative colitis (F54 plus K51.–); and urticaria (F54 plus L50.–).

Includes: psychological factors affecting physical conditions
Excludes: tension-type headache (G44.2)

F55   Abuse of non-dependence-producing substances

A wide variety of medicaments, proprietary drugs, and folk remedies may be involved, but three particularly important groups are: psychotropic drugs that do not produce dependence, such as antidepressants; laxatives; and analgesics that can be purchased without medical prescription, such as aspirin and paracetamol. Although the medication may have been medically prescribed or recommended in the first instance, prolonged, unnecessary, and often excessive dosage develops, which is facilitated by the availability of the substances without medical prescription.

Persistent and unjustified use of these substances is usually associated with unnecessary expense, often involves unnecessary contacts with medical professionals or supporting staff, and is sometimes marked by the harmful physical effects of the substances. Attempts to discourage or forbid the use of the substances are often met with resistance; for laxatives and analgesics this may be in spite of warnings about (or even the development of) physical problems such as renal dysfunction or electrolyte disturbances. Although it is usually clear that the patient has a strong motivation to take the substance, there is no development of dependence (F1x.2) or withdrawal symptoms (F1x.3) as in the case of the psychoactive substances specified in F10–F19.

A fourth character may be used to identify the type of substance involved.

F55.0   Antidepressants
(such as tricyclic and tetracyclic antidepressants and monamine oxidase inhibitors)

F55.1   Laxatives

F55.2   Analgesics
(such as aspirin, paracetamol, phenacetin, not specified as psycho-active in F10–F19)

F55.3   Antacids

F55.4   Vitamins

F55.5   Steroids or hormones

F55.6   Specific herbal or folk remedies

F55.8   Other substances that do not produce dependence
(such as diuretics)

F55.9   Unspecified
Excludes: abuse of (dependence-producing) psychoactive substance (F10–F19)

F59   Unspecified behavioural syndromes associated with physiological disturbances and physical factors

Includes: psychogenic physiological dysfunction NOS

One

F65   Disorders of sexual preference
    F65.0   Fetishism
    F65.1   Fetishistic transvestism
    F65.2   Exhibitionism
    F65.3   Voyeurism
    F65.4   Pædophilia
    F65.5   Sadomasochism
    F65.6   Multiple disorders of sexual preference
    F65.8   Other disorders of sexual preference
    F65.9   Disorder of sexual preference, unspecified

F66   Psychological and behavioural disorders associated with sexual development and orientation
    F66.0   Sexual maturation disorder
    F66.1   Egodystonic sexual orientation
    F66.2   Sexual relationship disorder
    F66.8   Other psychosexual development disorders
    F66.9   Psychosexual development disorder, unspecified

A fifth character may be used to indicate association with:
    ..x0 Heterosexuality
    ..x1 Homosexuality
    ..x2 Bisexuality
    ..x8 Other, including prepubertal

F68   Other disorders of adult personality and behaviour
    F68.0   Elaboration of physical symptoms for psychological reasons
    F68.1   Intentional production or feigning of symptoms or disabilities either physical or psychological [factitious disorder]
    F68.8   Other specified disorders of adult personality and behaviour

F69   Unspecified disorder of adult personality and behaviour

Introduction

This block includes a variety of clinically significant conditions and behaviour patterns which tend to be persistent and are the expression of an individual's characteristic lifestyle and mode of relating to self and others. Some of these conditions and patterns of behaviour emerge early in the course of individual development, as a result of both constitutional factors and social experience, while others are acquired later in life.

One

F60–F62 Specific personality disorders, mixed and other personality disorders, and enduring personality changes

These types of condition comprise deeply ingrained and enduring behaviour patterns, manifesting themselves as inflexible responses to a broad range of personal and social situations. They represent either extreme or significant deviations from the way the average individual in a given culture perceives, thinks, feels, and particularly relates to others. Such behaviour patterns tend to be stable and to encompass multiple domains of behaviour and psychological functioning. They are frequently, but not always, associated with various degrees of subjective distress and problems in social functioning and performance.

Personality disorders differ from personality change in their timing and the mode of their emergence: they are developmental conditions, which appear in childhood or adolescence and continue into adulthood. They are not secondary to another mental disorder or brain disease, although they may precede and coexist with other disorders. In contrast, personality change is acquired, usually during adult life, following severe or prolonged stress, extreme environmental deprivation, serious psychiatric disorder, or brain disease or injury (see F07.–).

Each of the conditions in this group can be classified according to its predominant behavioural manifestations. However, classification in this area is currently limited to the description of a series of types and subtypes, which are not mutually exclusive and which overlap in some of their characteristics.

Personality disorders are therefore subdivided according to clusters of traits that correspond to the most frequent or conspicuous behavioural manifestations. The subtypes so described are widely recognized as major forms of personality deviation. In making a diagnosis of personality disorder, the clinician should consider all aspects of personal functioning, although the diagnostic formulation, to be simple and efficient, will refer to only those dimensions or traits for which the suggested thresholds for severity are reached.

The assessment should be based on as many sources of information as possible. Although it is sometimes possible to evaluate a personality condition in a single interview with the patient, it is often necessary to have more than one interview and to collect history data from informants.

Cyclothymia and schizotypal disorders were formerly classified with the personality disorders but are now listed elsewhere (cyclothymia in F30–F39 and schizotypal disorder in F20–F29), since they seem to have many aspects in common with the other disorders in those blocks (e.g. phenomena, family history).

The subdivision of personality change is based on the cause or antecedent of such change, i.e. catastrophic experience, prolonged stress or strain, and psychiatric illness (excluding residual schizophrenia, which is classified under F20.5).

It is important to separate personality conditions from the disorders included in other categories of this book. If a personality condition precedes or follows a time-limited or chronic psychiatric disorder, both should be diagnosed.

Cultural or regional variations in the manifestations of personality conditions are important, but specific knowledge in this area is still scarce. Personality conditions that appear to be frequently recognized in a given part of the world but do not correspond to any one of the specified subtypes below may be classified as 'other' personality disorders and identified through a five-character code provided in an adaptation of this classification for that particular country or region. Local variations in the manifestations of a personality disorder may also be reflected in the wording of the diagnostic guidelines set for such conditions.

F60   Specific personality disorders

A specific personality disorder is a severe disturbance in the characterological constitution and behavioural tendencies of the individual, usually involving several areas of the personality, and nearly always associated with considerable personal and social disruption. Personality disorder tends to appear in late childhood or adolescence and continues to be manifest into adulthood. It is therefore unlikely that the diagnosis of personality disorder will be appropriate before the age of 16 or 17 years. General diagnostic guidelines applying to all personality disorders are presented below; supplementary descriptions are provided with each of the subtypes.

Diagnostic guidelines

Conditions not directly attributable to gross brain damage or disease, or to another psychiatric disorder, meeting the following criteria:

(a)   markedly disharmonious attitudes and behaviour, involving usually several areas of functioning, e.g. affectivity, arousal, impulse control, ways of perceiving and thinking, and style of relating to others;

(b)   the abnormal behaviour pattern is enduring, of long standing, and not limited to episodes of mental illness;

One

(c)   the abnormal behaviour pattern is pervasive and clearly maladaptive to a broad range of personal and social situations;

(d)   the above manifestations always appear during childhood or adolescence and continue into adulthood;

(e)   the disorder leads to considerable personal distress but this may only become apparent late in its course;

(f)   the disorder is usually, but not invariably, associated with significant problems in occupational and social performance.

For different cultures it may be necessary to develop specific sets of criteria with regard to social norms, rules and obligations. For diagnosing most of the subtypes listed below, clear evidence is usually required of the presence of *at least three* of the traits or behaviours given in the clinical description.

F60.0   *Paranoid personality disorder*
Personality disorder characterized by:

(a)   excessive sensitiveness to setbacks and rebuffs;

(b)   tendency to bear grudges persistently, e.g. refusal to forgive insults and injuries or slights;

(c)   suspiciousness and a pervasive tendency to distort experience by misconstruing the neutral or friendly actions of others as hostile or contemptuous;

(d)   a combative and tenacious sense of personal rights out of keeping with the actual situation;

(e)   recurrent suspicions, without justification, regarding sexual fidelity of spouse or sexual partner;

(f)   tendency to experience excessive self-importance, manifest in a persistent self-referential attitude;

(g)   preoccupation with unsubstantiated 'conspiratorial' explanations of events both immediate to the patient and in the world at large.

Includes: expansive paranoid, fanatic, querulant and sensitive paranoid personality (disorder)
Excludes: delusional disorder (F22.–)
          schizophrenia (F20.–)

F60.1   *Schizoid personality disorder*
Personality disorder meeting the following description:

(a)   few, if any, activities, provide pleasure;

(b)   emotional coldness, detachment or flattened affectivity;

(c)   limited capacity to express either warm, tender feelings or anger towards others;

(d)   apparent indifference to either praise or criticism;

(e)   little interest in having sexual experiences with another person (taking into account age);

(f)   almost invariable preference for solitary activities;

(g)   excessive preoccupation with fantasy and introspection;

(h)   lack of close friends or confiding relationships (or having only one) and of desire for such relationships;

(i)   marked insensitivity to prevailing social norms and conventions.

Excludes: Asperger's syndrome (F84.5)
delusional disorder (F22.0)
schizoid disorder of childhood (F84.5)
schizophrenia (F20.–)
schizotypal disorder (F21)

F60.2   *Dissocial personality disorder*

Personality disorder, usually coming to attention because of a gross disparity between behaviour and the prevailing social norms, and characterized by:

(a)   callous unconcern for the feelings of others;

(b)   gross and persistent attitude of irresponsibility and disregard for social norms, rules and obligations;

(c)   incapacity to maintain enduring relationships, though having no difficulty in establishing them;

(d)   very low tolerance to frustration and a low threshold for discharge of aggression, including violence;

(e)   incapacity to experience guilt or to profit from experience, particularly punishment;

(f)   marked proneness to blame others, or to offer plausible rationalizations, for the behaviour that has brought the patient into conflict with society.

There may also be persistent irritability as an associated feature. Conduct disorder during childhood and adolescence, though not invariably present, may further support the diagnosis.

Includes: amoral, antisocial, asocial, psychopathic, and sociopathic personality (disorder)

Excludes: conduct disorders (F91.–)
emotionally unstable personality disorder (F60.3)

F60.3   Emotionally unstable personality disorder

A personality disorder in which there is a marked tendency to act impulsively without consideration of the consequences, together with affective instability. The ability to plan ahead may be minimal, and outbursts of intense anger may often lead to violence or 'behavioural explosions'; these are easily precipitated when impulsive acts are criticized or thwarted by others. Two variants of this personality disorder are specified, and both share this general theme of impulsiveness and lack of self-control.

F60.30   Impulsive type

The predominant characteristics are emotional instability and lack of impulse control. Outbursts of violence or threatening behaviour are common, particularly in response to criticism by others.

Includes: explosive and aggressive personality (disorder)
Excludes: dissocial personality disorder (F60.2)

F60.31   Borderline type

Several of the characteristics of emotional instability are present; in addition, the patient's own self-image, aims, and internal preferences (including sexual) are often unclear or disturbed. There are usually chronic feelings of emptiness. A liability to become involved in intense and unstable relationships may cause repeated emotional crises and may be associated with excessive efforts to avoid abandonment and a series of suicidal threats or acts of self-harm (although these may occur without obvious precipitants).

Includes: borderline personality (disorder)

F60.4   Histrionic personality disorder

Personality disorder characterized by:

(a)   self-dramatization, theatricality, exaggerated expression of emotions;
(b)   suggestibility, easily influenced by others or by circumstances;
(c)   shallow and labile affectivity;
(d)   continual seeking for excitement and activities in which the patient is the centre of attention;
(e)   inappropriate seductiveness in appearance or behaviour;
(f)   over-concern with physical attractiveness.

Associated features may include egocentricity, self-indulgence, continuous longing for appreciation, feelings that are easily hurt, and persistent manipulative behaviour to achieve own needs.

Includes: hysterical and psychoinfantile personality (disorder)

F60.5   *Anankastic personality disorder*
Personality disorder characterized by:

(a)   feelings of excessive doubt and caution;

(b)   preoccupation with details, rules, lists, order, organization or schedule;

(c)   perfectionism that interferes with task completion;

(d)   excessive conscientiousness, scrupulousness, and undue preoccupation with productivity to the exclusion of pleasure and interpersonal relationships;

(e)   excessive pedantry and adherence to social conventions;

(f)   rigidity and stubbornness;

(g)   unreasonable insistence by the patient that others submit to exactly his or her way of doing things, or unreasonable reluctance to allow others to do things;

(h)   intrusion of insistent and unwelcome thoughts or impulses.

Includes: compulsive and obsessional personality (disorder)
              obsessive-compulsive personality disorder
Excludes: obsessive-compulsive disorder (F42.–)

F60.6   *Anxious [avoidant] personality disorder*
Personality disorder characterized by:

(a)   persistent and pervasive feelings of tension and apprehension;

(b)   belief that one is socially inept, personally unappealing, or inferior to others;

(c)   excessive preoccupation with being criticized or rejected in social situations;

(d)   unwillingness to become involved with people unless certain of being liked;

(e)   restrictions in lifestyle because of need to have physical security;

(f)   avoidance of social or occupational activities that involve significant interpersonal contact because of fear of criticism, disapproval, or rejection.

Associated features may include hypersensitivity to rejection and criticism.

F60.7   *Dependent personality disorder*
Personality disorder characterized by:

(a)   encouraging or allowing others to make most of one's important life decisions;

(b) subordination of one's own needs to those of others on whom one is dependent, and undue compliance with their wishes;

(c) unwillingness to make even reasonable demands on the people one depends on;

(d) feeling uncomfortable or helpless when alone, because of exaggerated fears of inability to care for oneself;

(e) preoccupation with fears of being abandoned by a person with whom one has a close relationship, and of being left to care for oneself;

(f) limited capacity to make everyday decisions without an excessive amount of advice and reassurance from others.

Associated features may include perceiving oneself as helpless, incompetent, and lacking stamina.

Includes: asthenic, inadequate, passive, and self-defeating personality (disorder)

F60.8 Other specific personality disorders

A personality disorder that fits none of the specific rubrics F60.0–F60.7.

Includes: eccentric, 'haltlose' type, immature, narcissistic, passive-aggressive, and psychoneurotic personality (disorder)

F60.9 Personality disorder, unspecified

Includes: character neurosis NOS

pathological personality NOS

F61 Mixed and other personality disorders

This category is intended for personality disorders and abnormalities that are often troublesome but do not demonstrate the specific patterns of symptoms that characterize the disorders described in F60.–. As a result they are often more difficult to diagnose than the disorders in that category. Two types are specified here by the fourth character; any other different types should be coded as F60.8.

F61.0 Mixed personality disorders

With features of several of the disorders in F60.– but without a predominant set of symptoms that would allow a more specific diagnosis.

F61.1 Troublesome personality changes

Not classifiable in F60.– or F62.– and regarded as secondary to a main diagnosis of a coexisting affective or anxiety disorder.

Excludes: accentuation of personality traits (Z73.1)

F62 Enduring personality changes, not attributable to brain damage and disease

Disorders of adult personality and behaviour that have developed in persons with no previous personality disorder following exposure to catastrophic or excessive prolonged stress, or following a severe psychiatric illness. These diagnoses should be made only when there is evidence of a definite and enduring change in a person's pattern of perceiving, relating to, or thinking about the environment and himself or herself. The personality change should be significant and be associated with inflexible and maladaptive behaviour not present before the pathogenic experience. The change should not be a direct manifestation of another mental disorder or a residual symptom of any antecedent mental disorder.

Excludes: personality and behavioural disorder due to brain damage or disease, damage and dysfunction (07.-)

F62.0 *Enduring personality change after catastrophic experience*
Enduring personality change, present for at least two years, following exposure to catastrophic stress. The stress must be so extreme that it is not necessary to consider personal vulnerability in order to explain its profound effect on the personality. The disorder is characterized by a hostile or distrustful attitude toward the world, social withdrawal, feelings of emptiness or hopelessness, a chronic feeling of 'being on edge' as if constantly threatened, and estrangement. Post-traumatic stress disorder (43.1) may precede this type of personality change.

Includes:
Personality change after:
> . concentration camp experiences
> . disasters
> . prolonged:
>> . captivity with an imminent possibility of being killed
>> . exposure to life-threatening situations such as being a victim of terrorism
> . torture

Excludes: post-traumatic stress disorder (43.1)

F62.1   *Enduring personality change after psychiatric illness*

Personality change, persisting for at least two years, attributable to the traumatic experience of suffering from a severe psychiatric illness. The change
cannot be explained by a previous personality disorder and should be differentiated from residual schizophrenia and other states of incomplete
recovery from an antecedent mental disorder. This disorder is characterized
by an excessive dependence on and a demanding attitude towards others;
conviction of being changed or stigmatized by the illness, leading to an
inability to form and maintain close and confiding personal relationships
and to social isolation; passivity, reduced interests, and diminished involvement in leisure activities; persistent complaints of being ill, which may be
associated with hypochondriacal claims and illness behaviour; dysphoric or
labile mood, not due to the presence of a current mental disorder or
antecedent mental disorder with residual affective symptoms; and long-
standing problems in social and occupational functioning.

F62.8   *Other enduring personality changes*

Chronic pain personality syndrome

F62.9   *Enduring personality change, unspecified*

F63   Habit and impulse disorders

This category includes certain behavioural disorders that are not classifiable under other rubrics. They are characterized by repeated acts that
have no clear rational motivation and that generally harm the patient's
own interests and those of other people. The patient reports that the
behaviour is associated with impulses to action that cannot be controlled. The causes of these conditions are not understood; the disorders
are grouped together because of broad descriptive similarities, not
because they are known to share any other important features. By con-
vention, the habitual excessive use of alcohol or drugs (F10–F19) and
impulse and habit disorders involving sexual (F65.–) or eating (F52.–)
behaviour are excluded.

F63.0   *Pathological gambling*

The disorder consists of frequent, repeated episodes of gambling that
dominate the individual's life to the detriment of social, occupational,
material, and family values and commitments.

Those who suffer from this disorder may put their jobs at risk, acquire large debts, and lie or break the law to obtain money or evade payment of debts. They describe an intense urge to gamble, which is difficult to control, together with preoccupation with ideas and images of the act of gambling and the circumstances that surround the act. These preoccupations and urges often increase at times when life is stressful.

This disorder is also called 'compulsive gambling' but this term is less appropriate because the behaviour is not compulsive in the technical sense, nor is the disorder related to obsessive-compulsive neurosis.

Diagnostic guidelines
The essential feature of the disorder is persistently repeated gambling, which continues and often increases despite adverse social consequences such as impoverishment, impaired family relationships, and disruption of personal life.

Includes: compulsive gambling

Differential diagnosis
Pathological gambling should be distinguished from:

(a)   gambling and betting (F99.2) (frequent gambling for excitement, or in an attempt to make money; people in this category are likely to curb their habit when confronted with heavy losses, or other adverse effects);

(b)   excessive gambling by manic patients (F30.–);

(c)   gambling by sociopathic personalities (F60.2) (in which there is a wider persistent disturbance of social behaviour, shown in acts that are aggressive or in other ways demonstrate a marked lack of concern for the well-being and feelings of other people).

F63.1   Pathological fire-setting [pyromania]
The disorder is characterized by multiple acts of, or attempts at, setting fire to property or other objects, without apparent motive, and by a persistent preoccupation with subjects related to fire and burning. There may also be an abnormal interest in fire-engines and other fire-fighting equipment, in other associations of fires, and in calling out the fire service.

Diagnostic guidelines
The essential features are:

(a)   repeated fire-setting without any obvious motive such as monetary gain, revenge, or political extremism;

(b)   an intense interest in watching fires burn; and
(c)   reported feelings of increasing tension before the act, and intense excite-
       ment immediately after it has been carried out.

Differential diagnosis

Pathological fire-setting should be distinguished from:

(a)   deliberate fire-setting without a manifest psychiatric disorder (in these
       cases there is an obvious motive) (F99.2, observation for suspected men-
       tal disorder);
(b)   fire-setting by a young person with conduct disorder (F91.1), where
       there is evidence of other disordered behaviour such as stealing, aggres-
       sion, or truancy;
(c)   fire-setting by an adult with sociopathic personality disorder (F60.2),
       where there is evidence of other persistent disturbance of social behav-
       iour such as aggression, or other indications of lack of concern with the
       interests and feelings of other people;
(d)   fire-setting in schizophrenia (F20.–), when fires are typically started in
       response to delusional ideas or commands from hallucinated voices;
(e)   fire-setting in organic psychiatric disorders (F00–F09), when fires are
       started accidentally as a result of confusion, poor memory, or lack of
       awareness of the consequences of the act, or a combination of these fac-
       tors.

Dementia or acute organic states may also lead to inadvertent fire-setting; acute drunkenness, chronic alcoholism or other drug intoxication
(F10–F19) are other causes.

F63.2   Pathological stealing [kleptomania]

The disorder is characterized by repeated failure to resist impulses to
steal objects that are not acquired for personal use or monetary gain. The
objects may instead be discarded, given away, or hoarded.

Diagnostic guidelines

There is an increasing sense of tension before, and a sense of gratification during and immediately after, the act. Although some effort at concealment is usually made, not all the opportunities for this are taken. The
theft is a solitary act, not carried out with an accomplice. The individual
may express anxiety, despondency, and guilt between episodes of stealing from shops (or other premises) but this does not prevent repetition.

Cases meeting this description alone, and not secondary to one of the disorders listed below, are uncommon.

Differential diagnosis
Pathological stealing should be distinguished from:

(a) recurrent shoplifting without a manifest psychiatric disorder, when the acts are more carefully planned, and there is an obvious motive of personal gain (F99.2, observation for suspected mental disorder);

(b) organic mental disorder (F00–F09), when there is recurrent failure to pay for goods as a consequence of poor memory and other kinds of intellectual deterioration;

(c) depressive disorder with stealing (F30–F33); some depressed individuals steal, and may do so repeatedly as long as the depressive disorder persists.

F63.3 Trichotillomania
A disorder characterized by noticeable hair loss due to a recurrent failure to resist impulses to pull out hairs. The hair-pulling is usually preceded by mounting tension and is followed by a sense of relief or gratification. This diagnosis should not be made if there is a pre-existing inflammation of the skin, or if the hair-pulling is in response to a delusion or a hallucination.

Excludes: stereotyped movement disorder with hair-plucking (F98.4)

F63.8 Other habit and impulse disorders
This category should be used for other kinds of persistently repeated maladaptive behaviour that are not secondary to a recognized psychiatric syndrome, and in which it appears that there is repeated failure to resist impulses to carry out the behaviour. There is a prodromal period of tension with a feeling of release at the time of the act.

Includes: intermittent explosive (behaviour) disorder

F63.9 Habit and impulse disorder, unspecified

F64 Gender identity disorders

F64.0 Transsexualism

F64.1   *Dual-role transvestism*

F64.2   *Gender identity disorder of childhood*

Disorders, usually first manifest during early childhood (and always well before puberty), characterized by a persistent and intense distress about assigned sex, together with a desire to be (or insistence that one is) of the other sex. There is a persistent preoccupation with the dress and/or activities of the opposite sex and/or repudiation of the patient's own sex. These disorders are thought to be relatively uncommon and should not be confused with the much more frequent nonconformity with stereotypic sex-role behaviour. The diagnosis of gender identity disorder in childhood requires a profound disturbance of the normal sense of maleness or femaleness; mere 'tomboyishness' in girls or 'girlish' behaviour in boys is not sufficient. The diagnosis cannot be made when the individual has reached puberty.

Because gender identity disorder of childhood has many features in common with the other identity disorders in this section, it has been classified in F64.– rather than in F90–F98.

Diagnostic guidelines

The essential diagnostic feature is the child's pervasive and persistent desire to be (or insistence that he or she is of) the opposite sex to that assigned, together with an intense rejection of the behaviour, attributes, and/or attire of the assigned sex. Typically, this is first manifest during the preschool years; for the diagnosis to be made, the disorder must have been apparent before puberty. In both sexes, there may be repudiation of the anatomical structures of their own sex, but this is an uncommon, probably rare, manifestation. Characteristically, children with a gender identity disorder deny being disturbed by it, although they may be distressed by the conflict with the expectations of their family or peers and by the teasing and/or rejection to which they may be subjected.

More is known about these disorders in boys than in girls. Typically, from the preschool years onwards, boys are preoccupied with types of play and other activities stereotypically associated with females, and there may often be a preference for dressing in girls' or women's clothes. However, such cross-dressing does not cause sexual excitement (unlike fetishistic transvestism in adults (F65.1)). They may have a very strong desire to participate in the games and pastimes of girls, female dolls are often their favourite toys, and girls are regularly their preferred playmates. Social ostracism tends to arise during the early years of schooling and is often at a peak in middle childhood, with humiliating teasing by other boys. Grossly feminine behaviour may lessen during early adolescence but follow-up studies indicate that between one-third and two-thirds of boys with gender identity disorder of childhood show a homosexual orientation during and after adolescence. However, very few exhibit transsexualism in adult life (although most adults with transsexualism report having had a gender identity problem in childhood).

In clinic samples, gender identity disorders are less frequent in girls than in boys, but it is not known whether this sex ratio applies in the general population. In girls, as in boys, there is usually an early manifestation of a preoccupation with behaviour stereotypically associated with the opposite sex. Typically, girls with these disorders have male companions and show an avid interest in sports and rough-and-tumble play; they lack interest in dolls and in taking female roles in make-believe games such as 'mothers and fathers' or playing 'house'. Girls with a gender identity disorder tend not to experience the same degree of social ostracism as boys, although they may suffer from teasing in later childhood or adolescence. Most give up an exaggerated insistence on male activities and attire as they approach adolescence, but some retain a male identification and go on to show a homosexual orientation.

Rarely, a gender identity disorder may be associated with a persistent repudiation of the anatomic structures of the assigned sex. In girls, this may be manifest by repeated assertions that they have, or will grow, a penis, by rejection of urination in the sitting position, or by the assertion that they do not want to grow breasts or to menstruate. In boys, it may be shown by repeated assertions that they will grow up physically to become a woman, that penis and testes are disgusting or will disappear, and/or that it would be better not to have a penis or testes.

Excludes: egodystonic sexual orientation (F66.1)
sexual maturation disorder (F66.0)

F64.8   *Other gender identity disorders*

F64.9   *Gender identity disorder, unspecified*

F65   Disorders of sexual preference

F65.0   *Fetishism*

F65.1   *Fetishistic transvestism*

F65.2   *Exhibitionism*

F65.3   *Voyeurism*

F65.4   *Pædophilia*

F65.5   *Sadomasochism*

F65.6   *Multiple disorders of sexual preference*

F65.8   *Other disorders of sexual preference*

F65.9   *Disorder of sexual preference, unspecified*

F66   Psychological and behavioural disorders associated with sexual development and orientation

Note: Sexual orientation alone is not to be regarded as a disorder.

The following five-character codes may be used to indicate variations of sexual development or orientation that may be problematic for the individual:

F66.x0 Heterosexual

F66.x1 Homosexual

F66.x2 Bisexual
To be used only when there is clear evidence of sexual attraction to members of both sexes.

F66.x8 Other, including prepubertal

F66.0   *Sexual maturation disorder*
The individual suffers from uncertainty about his or her gender identity or sexual orientation, which causes anxiety or depression. Most commonly this occurs in adolescents who are not certain whether they are homosexual, heterosexual, or bisexual in orientation, or in individuals

who after a period of apparently stable sexual orientation, often within a long-standing relationship, find that their sexual orientation is changing.

F66.1   *Egodystonic sexual orientation*
The gender identity or sexual preference is not in doubt but the individual wishes it were different because of associated psychological and behavioural disorders and may seek treatment in order to change it.

F66.2   *Sexual relationship disorder*
The gender identity or sexual preference abnormality is responsible for difficulties in forming or maintaining a relationship with a sexual partner.

F66.8   *Other psychosexual development disorders*

F66.9   *Psychosexual development disorder, unspecified*

F68   **Other disorders of adult personality and behaviour**

F68.0   *Elaboration of physical symptoms for psychological reasons*

F68.1   *Intentional production or feigning of symptoms or disabilities, either physical or psychological [factitious disorder]*

F68.8   *Other specified disorders of adult personality and behaviour*

F69   **Unspecified disorder of adult personality and behaviour**

F99 Unspecified mental disorder and problems falling short of criteria for any specified mental disorder

F99.0[1] *Mental disorder, not otherwise specified*
Non-recommended residual category, when no other code from F00–F98 can be used.

F99.1[1] *Relationship problem, falling short of criteria for any specified mental disorder, but giving rise to clinical referral for assessment or service provision*
Difficulties in bedtime routines or in feeding in young children constitute examples of problems that should be coded here.

F99.2[1] *Emotional or behavioural problem, falling short of criteria for any specified mental disorder, but giving rise to clinical referral for assessment or service provision*
Undue shyness or temper tantrums constitute examples of problems that should be coded here.

---

[1] This four-character code is not included in Chapter V(F codes) of ICD-10.

Axis Two

Specific Disorders of Psychological Development

List of categories

Introduction

The disorders included in F80–F83 and F88-F89 have the following features in common:

(a)   an onset that is invariably during infancy or childhood;

---

[1]   F84, Pervasive developmental disorders, is included in Axis One, as explained in the Introduction to this book.

(b)   an impairment or delay in the development of functions that are strongly related to biological maturation of the central nervous system; and

(c)   a steady course that does not involve the remissions and relapses that tend to be characteristic of many mental disorders.

In most cases, the functions affected include language, visuo-spatial skills and/or motor coordination. It is characteristic for the impairments to lessen progressively as children grow older (although milder deficits often remain in adult life). Usually, the history is of a delay or impairment that has been present from as early as it could be reliably detected, with no prior period of normal development. Most of these conditions are several times more common in boys than in girls.

It is characteristic of developmental disorders that a family history of similar or related disorders is common, and there is presumptive evidence that genetic factors play an important role in the etiology of many (but not all) cases. Environmental factors often influence the developmental functions affected but in most cases they are not of paramount influence. However, although there is generally good agreement on the overall conceptualization of disorders in this section, the etiology in most cases is unknown and there is continuing uncertainty regarding both the boundaries and the precise subdivisions of developmental disorders.

F80   Specific developmental disorders of speech and language

These are disorders in which normal patterns of language acquisition are disturbed from the early stages of development. The conditions are not directly attributable to neurological or speech mechanism abnormalities, sensory impairments, mental retardation, or environmental factors. The child may be better able to communicate or understand in certain very familiar situations than in others, but language ability in every setting is impaired.

Differential diagnosis
As with other developmental disorders, the first difficulty in diagnosis concerns the differentiation from normal variations in development. Normal children vary widely in the age at which they first acquire spoken language and in the pace at which language skills become firmly established. Such normal variations are of little or no clinical significance, as the great majority of 'slow speakers' go on to develop entirely normally. In sharp contrast, children with specific developmental disor-

ders of speech and language, although most ultimately acquire a normal level of language skills, have multiple associated problems. Language delay is often followed by difficulties in reading and spelling, abnormalities in interpersonal relationships, and emotional and behavioural disorders. Accordingly, early and accurate diagnosis of specific developmental disorders of speech and language is important. There is no clear-cut demarcation from the extremes of normal variation, but four main criteria are useful in suggesting the occurrence of a clinically significant disorder: severity, course, pattern, and associated problems.

As a general rule, a language delay that is sufficiently severe to fall outside the limits of 2 standard deviations may be regarded as abnormal. Most cases of this severity have associated problems. The level of severity in statistical terms is of less diagnostic use in older children, however, because there is a natural tendency towards progressive improvement. In this situation the course provides a useful indicator. If the current level of impairment is mild but there is nevertheless a history of a previously severe degree of impairment, the likelihood is that the current functioning represents the sequelæ of a significant disorder rather than just normal variation. Attention should be paid to the pattern of speech and language functioning; if the pattern is abnormal (i.e. deviant and not just of a kind appropriate for an earlier phase of development), or if the child's speech or language includes qualitatively abnormal features, a clinically significant disorder is likely. Moreover, if a delay in some specific aspect of speech or language development is accompanied by scholastic deficits (such as specific retardation in reading or spelling), by abnormalities in interpersonal relationships, and/or by emotional or behavioural disturbance, the delay is unlikely to constitute just a normal variation.

The second difficulty in diagnosis concerns the differentiation from mental retardation or global developmental delay. Because intelligence includes verbal skills, it is likely that a child whose IQ is substantially below average will also show language development that is somewhat below average. The diagnosis of a specific developmental disorder implies that the specific delay is significantly out of keeping with the general level of cognitive functioning. Accordingly, when a language delay is simply part of a more pervasive mental retardation or global developmental delay, a mental retardation coding (F70–F79) using Axis Three should be used, *not* an F80.– coding. However, it is common for mental retardation to be associated with an uneven pattern of intellectual performance and especially with a degree of language impairment that is more severe than the retardation in nonverbal skills. When this disparity is of such a marked degree that it is evident in everyday functioning, a specific developmental disorder of speech and language should be coded *in addition to* a coding for mental retardation (F70–F79).

The third difficulty concerns the differentiation from a disorder secondary to severe deafness or to some specific neurological or other structural abnormality. Severe deafness in early childhood will almost always lead to a marked delay and distortion of language development; such conditions should *not* be included here, as they are a direct consequence of the hearing impairment. However, it is not uncommon for the more severe developmental disorders of receptive language to be accompanied by partial selective hearing impairments (especially of high frequencies). The guideline is to *exclude* these disorders from F80–F89 if the severity of hearing loss constitutes a sufficient explanation for the language delay, but to *include* them if partial hearing loss is a complicating factor but not a sufficient direct cause. However, a hard and fast distinction is impossible to make. A similar principle applies with respect to neurological abnormalities and structural defects. Thus, an articulation abnormality directly due to a cleft palate or to a dysarthria resulting from cerebral palsy would be excluded from this block. On the other hand, the presence of subtle neurological abnormalities that could not have directly caused the speech or language delay would not constitute a reason for exclusion.

F80.0   *Specific speech articulation disorder*

A specific developmental disorder in which the child's use of speech sounds is below the appropriate level for his or her mental age, but in which there is a normal level of language skills.

Diagnostic guidelines

The age of acquisition of speech sounds, and the order in which these sounds develop, show considerable individual variation.

Normal development

At the age of 4 years, errors in speech sound production are common, but the child is able to be understood easily by strangers. By the age of 6–7, most speech sounds will be acquired. Although difficulties may remain with certain sound combinations, these should not result in any problems of communication. By the age of 11–12 years, mastery of almost all speech sounds should be acquired.

Abnormal development

occurs when the child's acquisition of speech sounds is delayed and/or deviant, leading to: misarticulations in the child's speech with consequent difficulties for others in understanding him or her; omissions, distortions, or substitutions of speech sounds; and inconsistencies in the co-occurrence of sounds (i.e. the child may produce phonemes correctly in some word positions but not in others).

The diagnosis should be made only when the severity of the articulation disorder is outside the limits of normal variation for the child's mental age; nonverbal intelligence is within the normal range; expressive and receptive language skills are within the normal range; the articulation abnormalities are not directly attributable to a sensory, structural or neurological abnormality; and the mispronunciations are clearly abnormal in the context of colloquial usage in the child's subculture.

Includes: developmental articulation disorder
developmental phonological disorder
dyslalia
functional articulation disorder
lalling

Excludes: articulation disorder due to:
aphasia NOS (R47.0)
apraxia (R48.2)
articulation impairments associated with a developmental disorder of expressive or receptive language (F80.1, F80.2)
cleft palate or other structural abnormalities of the oral structures involved in speech (Q35–Q38)
hearing loss (H90–H91)
mental retardation (F70–F79)

F80.1 *Expressive language disorder*

A specific developmental disorder in which the child's ability to use expressive spoken language is markedly below the appropriate level for his or her mental age, but in which language comprehension is within normal limits. There may or may not be abnormalities in articulation.

Diagnostic guidelines

Although considerable individual variation occurs in normal language development, the absence of single words (or word approximations) by the age of 2 years, and the failure to generate simple two-word phrases by 3 years, should be taken as significant signs of delay. Later difficulties include: restricted vocabulary development; overuse of a small set of general words, difficulties in selecting appropriate words, and word substitutions; short utterance length; immature sentence structure; syntactical errors, especially *omissions* of word endings or prefixes; and misuse of or failure to use grammatical features such as prepositions, pronouns, articles, and verb and noun inflexions. Incorrect over-generalizations of rules may also occur, as may a lack of sentence fluency and difficulties in sequencing when recounting past events.

It is frequent for impairments in spoken language to be accompanied by delays or abnormalities in word-sound production.

The diagnosis should be made only when the severity of the delay in the development of expressive language is outside the limits of normal variation for the child's mental age, but receptive language skills are within normal limits (although they may often be somewhat below average). The use of nonverbal cues (such as smiles and gesture) and 'internal' language as reflected in imaginative or make-believe play should be relatively intact, and the ability to communicate socially without words should be relatively unimpaired. The child will seek to communicate in spite of the language impairment and will tend to compensate for lack of speech by use of demonstration, gesture, mime, or non-speech vocalizations. However, associated difficulties in peer relationships, emotional disturbance, behavioural disruption, and/or overactivity and inattention are not uncommon, particularly in school-age children. In a minority of cases there may be some associated partial (often selective) hearing loss, but this should not be of a severity sufficient to account for the language delay. Inadequate involvement in conversational interchanges, or more general environmental privation, may play a major or contributory role in the impaired development of expressive language. Where this is the case, the environmental causal factor should be noted by means of the appropriate code on Axis Five (Associated abnormal psychosocial situations). The impairment in spoken language should have been evident from infancy without any clear prolonged phase of normal language usage. However, a history of apparently normal first use of a *few* single words, followed by a setback or failure to progress, is not uncommon.

Includes: developmental dysphasia or aphasia, expressive type

Excludes: acquired aphasia with epilepsy [Landau-Kleffner syndrome] (F80.3)

            developmental aphasia or dysphasia, receptive type (F80.2)

dysphasia and aphasia NOS (R47.0)

elective mutism (F94.0)

mental retardation (F79–F79)

pervasive developmental disorders (F84.–)

F80.2   Receptive language disorder

A specific developmental disorder in which the child's understanding of language is below the appropriate level for his or her mental age. In almost all cases, expressive language is markedly disturbed and abnormalities in word-sound production are common.

Diagnostic guidelines

Failure to respond to familiar names (in the absence of nonverbal clues) by the first birthday, inability to identify at least a few common objects by 18 months, or failure to follow simple, routine instructions by the age of 2 years should be taken as significant signs of delay. Later difficulties include inability to understand grammatical structures (negatives, questions, comparatives, etc.), and lack of understanding of more subtle aspects of language (tone of voice, gesture, etc.).

The diagnosis should be made only when the severity of the delay in receptive language is outside the normal limits of variation for the child's mental age, and when the criteria for a pervasive developmental disorder are *not* met. In almost all cases, the development of expressive language is also severely delayed and abnormalities in word-sound production are common. Of all the varieties of specific developmental disorders of speech and language, this has the highest rate of associated socio-emotional–behavioural disturbance. Such disturbances do not take any specific form, but hyperactivity and inattention, social ineptness and isolation from peers, and anxiety, sensitivity, or undue shyness are all relatively frequent. Children with the most severe forms of receptive language impairment may be somewhat delayed in their social development, may echo language that they do not understand, and may show somewhat restricted interest patterns. However, they differ from autistic children in usually showing normal social reciprocity, normal make-believe play, normal use of parents for comfort, near-normal use of gesture, and only mild impairments in nonverbal communication. Some degree of high-frequency hearing loss is not infrequent, but the degree of deafness is not sufficient to account for the language impairment.

Includes: congenital auditory imperception

developmental aphasia or dysphasia, receptive type

developmental Wernicke's aphasia

word deafness

mixed receptive–expressive language disorder

Excludes: acquired aphasia with epilepsy [Landau–Kleffner syndrome] (F80.3)

autism (F84.0, F84.1)

dysphasia and aphasia, NOS (R47.0) or expressive type (F80.1)

elective mutism (F94.0)

language delay due to deafness (H90–H91)

mental retardation (F70–F79)

F80.3   *Acquired aphasia with epilepsy [Landau-Kleffner syndrome]*

A disorder in which the child, having previously made normal progress in language development, loses both receptive and expressive language skills but retains general intelligence. Onset of the disorder is accompanied by paroxysmal abnormalities on the EEG (almost always from the temporal lobes, usually bilateral, but often with more widespread disturbance), and in the majority of cases also by epileptic seizures. Typically the onset is between the ages of 3 and 7 years but the disorder can arise earlier or later in childhood. In a quarter of cases the loss of language occurs gradually over a period of some months, but more often the loss is abrupt, with skills being lost over days or weeks. The temporal association between onset of seizures and loss of language is rather variable, with either one preceding the other by a few months to 2 years. It is highly characteristic that the impairment of receptive language is profound, with difficulties in auditory comprehension often being the first manifestation of the condition. Some children become mute, some are restricted to jargon-like sounds, and some show milder deficits in word fluency and output often accompanied by misarticulations. In a few cases voice quality is affected, with a loss of normal inflexions. Sometimes language functions appear fluctuating in the early phases of the disorder. Behavioural and emotional disturbances are quite common in the months after the initial language loss, but they tend to improve as the child acquires some means of communication.

The etiology of the condition is not known but the clinical characteristics suggest the possibility of an inflammatory encephalitic process. The course of the disorder is quite variable: about two-thirds of the children are left with a more or less severe receptive language deficit and about a third make a complete recovery.

Excludes: acquired aphasia due to cerebral trauma, tumour or other known disease process

autism (F84.0, F84.1)

other disintegrative disorder of childhood (F84.3)

F80.8 *Other developmental disorders of speech and language*

Includes: lisping

F80.9 *Developmental disorder of speech and language, unspecified*

This category should be avoided as far as possible and should be used only for unspecified disorders in which there is significant impairment in the development of speech or language that cannot be accounted for by mental retardation, or by neurological, sensory or physical impairments that directly affect speech or language.

Includes: language disorder NOS

F81   Specific developmental disorders of scholastic skills

The concept of specific developmental disorders of scholastic skills is directly comparable to that of specific developmental disorders of speech and language (see F80.–) and essentially the same issues of definition and measurement apply. These are disorders in which the normal patterns of skill acquisition are disturbed from the early stages of development. They are not simply a consequence of a lack of opportunity to learn, nor are they due to any form of acquired brain trauma or disease. Rather, the disorders are thought to stem from abnormalities in cognitive processing that derive largely from some type of biological dysfunction. As with most other developmental disorders, the conditions are substantially more common in boys than in girls.

Five kinds of difficulty arise in diagnosis. First, there is the need to differentiate the disorders from normal variations in scholastic achievement. The considerations are similar to those in language disorders, and the same criteria are proposed for the assessment of abnormality (with the necessary modifications that arise from evaluation of scholastic achievement rather than language). Second, there is the need to take developmental course into account. This is important for two different reasons:

(a)   Severity: the significance of one year's retardation in reading at age 7 years is quite different from that of one year's retardation at 14 years.

(b)   Change in pattern: it is common for a language delay in the preschool years to resolve so far as spoken language is concerned but to be followed by a specific reading retardation which, in turn, diminishes in adolescence; the principal problem remaining in early adulthood is a severe spelling disorder. The condition is the same throughout but the pattern alters with increasing age; the diagnostic criteria need to take into account this developmental change.

Third, there is the difficulty that scholastic skills have to be taught and learned: they are *not* simply a function of biological maturation. Inevitably a child's level of skills will depend on family circumstances and schooling, as well as on his or her own individual characteristics. Unfortunately, there is no straightforward and unambiguous way of differentiating scholastic difficulties due to lack of adequate experiences from those due to some individual disorder. There are good reasons for supposing that the distinction is real and clinically valid but the diagnosis in individual cases is difficult. Fourth, although research findings provide support for the hypothesis of underlying abnormalities in cognitive processing, there is no easy way in the individual child to differentiate those that *cause* reading difficulties from those that derive from or are associated with poor reading skills. The difficulty is compounded by the finding that reading disorders may stem from more than one type of cognitive abnormality. Fifth, there are continuing uncertainties over the best way of subdividing the specific developmental disorders of scholastic skills.

Children learn to read, write, spell, and perform arithmetical computations when they are introduced to these activities at home and at school. Countries vary widely in the age at which formal schooling is started, in the syllabus followed within schools, and hence in the skills that children are expected to have acquired by different ages. This disparity of expectations is greater during elementary or primary school years (i.e. up to age about 11 years) and complicates the issue of devising operational definitions of disorders of scholastic skills that have cross-national validity.

Nevertheless, within all education settings, it is clear that each chronological age group of schoolchildren contains a wide spread of scholastic attainments and that some children are underachieving in specific aspects of attainment relative to their general level of intellectual functioning.

Specific developmental disorders of scholastic skills (SDDSS) comprise groups of disorders manifested by specific and significant impairments in learning of scholastic skills. These impairments in learning are not the direct result of other disorders (such as mental retardation, gross neurological deficits, uncorrected visual or auditory problems, or emotional disturbances), although they may occur concurrently with such conditions. SDDSS frequently occur in conjunction with other clinical syndromes (such as attention deficit disorder or conduct disorder) or other developmental disorders (such as specific developmental disorder of motor function or specific developmental disorders of speech and language).

The etiology of SDDSS is not known, but there is an assumption of the primacy of biological factors that interact with nonbiological factors (such as opportunity for learning and quality of teaching) to produce the manifestations. Although these disorders are related to biological maturation, there is no implication that children with these disorders are simply at the lower end of a normal continuum and will therefore 'catch up' with time. In many instances, traces of these disorders may continue through adolescence into adulthood. Nevertheless, it is a necessary diagnostic feature that the disorders were manifest in some form during the early years of schooling. Children can fall behind in their scholastic performance at a later stage in their educational careers (because of lack of interest, poor teaching, emotional disturbance, an increase or change in pattern of task demands, etc.), but such problems do not form part of the concept of SDDSS.

Diagnostic guidelines

There are several basic requirements for the diagnosis of any of the specific developmental disorders of scholastic skills. First, there must be a clinically significant degree of impairment in the specified scholastic skill. This may be judged on the basis of severity as defined in scholastic terms (i.e. a degree that may be expected to occur in less than 3% of schoolchildren); on developmental precursors (i.e. the scholastic difficulties were preceded by developmental delays or deviance – most often in speech or language – in the preschool years); on associated problems (such as inattention, overactivity, emotional disturbance, or conduct difficulties); on pattern (i.e. the presence of qualitative abnormalities that are not usually part of normal development); and on response (i.e. the scholastic difficulties do not rapidly and readily remit with increased help at home and/or at school).

Second, the impairment must be specific in the sense that it is not solely explained by mental retardation or by lesser impairments in gen-

Two

eral intelligence. Because IQ and scholastic achievement do not run exactly in parallel, this distinction can be made only on the basis of individually administered standardized tests of achievement and IQ that are appropriate for the relevant culture and educational system. Such tests should be used in connection with statistical tables that provide data on the average expected level of achievement for any given IQ level at any given chronological age. This last requirement is necessary because of the importance of statistical regression effects: diagnoses based on subtractions of achievement age from mental age are bound to be seriously misleading. In routine clinical practice, however, it is unlikely that these requirements will be met in most instances. Accordingly, the clinical guideline is simply that the child's level of attainment must be very substantially below that expected for a child of the same mental age.

Third, the impairment must be developmental, in the sense that it must have been present during the early years of schooling and not acquired later in the educational process. The history of the child's school progress should provide evidence on this point.

Fourth, there must be no external factors that could provide a sufficient reason for the scholastic difficulties. As indicated above, a diagnosis of SDDSS should generally rest on positive evidence of clinically significant disorder of scholastic achievement associated with factors intrinsic to the child's development. To learn effectively, however, children must have adequate learning opportunities. Accordingly, if it is clear that the poor scholastic achievement is directly due to very prolonged school absence without teaching at home or to grossly inadequate education, the disorders should not be coded here. Frequent absences from school or educational discontinuities resulting from changes in school are usually *not* sufficient to give rise to scholastic retardation of the degree necessary for diagnosis of SDDSS. However, poor schooling may complicate or add to the problem, in which case the school factors may be coded in Axis Five.

Fifth, the SDDSS must not be *directly* due to uncorrected visual or hearing impairments.

Differential diagnosis

It is clinically important to differentiate between SDDSS that arise in the absence of any diagnosable neurological disorder and those that are secondary to some neurological condition such as cerebral palsy. In practice this differentiation is often difficult to make (because of the uncertain significance of multiple 'soft' neurological signs), and research findings do not show any clear-cut differentiation in either the pattern or course of SDDSS according to the presence or absence of overt neurological dysfunction. Accordingly, although this does *not* form part of the diagnostic criteria, it *is* necessary that the presence of any associated disorder be separately coded in the appropriate neurological section of the classification.

F81.0   *Specific reading disorder*

The main feature of this disorder is a specific and significant impairment in the development of reading skills, which is not solely accounted for by mental age, visual acuity problems, or inadequate schooling. Reading comprehension skill, reading word recognition, oral reading skill, and performance of tasks requiring reading may all be affected. Spelling difficulties are frequently associated with specific reading disorder and often remain into adolescence even after some progress in reading has been made. Children with specific reading disorder frequently have a history of specific developmental disorders of speech and language, and comprehensive assessment of current language functioning often reveals subtle contemporaneous difficulties. In addition to academic failure, poor school attendance and problems with social adjustment are frequent complications, particularly in the later elementary and secondary school years. The condition is found in all known languages, but there is uncertainty as to whether or not its frequency is affected by the nature of the language and of the written script.

Diagnostic guidelines

The child's reading performance should be significantly below the level expected on the basis of age, general intelligence, and school placement. Performance is best assessed by means of an individually administered, standardized test of reading accuracy and comprehension. The precise nature of the reading problem depends on the expected level of reading, and on the language and script. However, in the early stages of learning an alphabetic script, there may be difficulties in reciting the alphabet, in giving the correct names of letters, in giving simple rhymes for words, and in analysing or categorizing sounds (in spite of normal auditory acuity). Later, there may be errors in oral reading skills such as shown by:

(a)   omissions, substitutions, distortions, or additions of words or parts of words;

(b)   slow reading rate;

(c)   false starts, long hesitations or 'loss of place' in text, and inaccurate phrasing; and (d)　reversals of words in sentences or of letters within words.

There may also be deficits in reading comprehension, as shown by, for example:

(e)　an inability to recall facts read;
(f)　inability to draw conclusions or inferences from material read; and
(g)　use of general knowledge as background information rather than of information from a particular story to answer questions about a story read.

In later childhood and in adult life, it is common for spelling difficulties to be more profound than the reading deficits. It is characteristic that the spelling difficulties often involve phonetic errors, and it seems that both the reading and spelling problems may derive in part from an impairment in phonological analysis. Little is known about the nature or frequency of spelling errors in children who have to read non-phonetic languages, and little is known about the types of error in non-alphabetic scripts.

Specific developmental disorders of reading are commonly preceded by a history of disorders in speech or language development. In other cases, children may pass language milestones at the normal age but have difficulties in auditory processing as shown by problems in sound categorization, in rhyming, and possibly by deficits in speech sound discrimination, auditory sequential memory, and auditory association. In some cases, too, there may be problems in visual processing (such as in letter discrimination); however, these are common among children who are just beginning to learn to read and hence are probably not directly causally related to the poor reading. Difficulties in attention, often associated with overactivity and impulsivity, are also common. The precise pattern of developmental difficulties in the preschool period varies considerably from child to child, as does their severity; nevertheless such difficulties are usually (but not invariably) present.

Associated emotional and/or behavioural disturbances are also common during the school-age period. Emotional problems are more common during the early school years, but conduct disorders and hyperactivity syndromes are most likely to be present in later childhood and adolescence. Low self-esteem is common and problems in school adjustment and in peer relationships are also frequent.

Includes:　'backward reading'
　　　　　　developmental dyslexia

specific reading retardation
spelling difficulties associated with a reading disorder

Excludes: acquired alexia and dyslexia (R48.0)
acquired reading difficulties secondary to emotional disturbance (F93.–)
spelling disorder not associated with reading difficulties
(F81.1)

F81.1 *Specific spelling disorder*
The main feature of this disorder is a specific and significant impairment
in the development of spelling skills in the *absence* of a history of specific reading disorder, which is not solely accounted for by low mental
age, visual acuity problems, or inadequate schooling. The ability to spell
orally and to write out words correctly are both affected. Children whose
problem is solely one of handwriting should not be included, but in some
cases spelling difficulties may be associated with problems in writing.
Unlike the usual pattern of specific reading disorder, the spelling errors
tend to be predominantly phonetically accurate.

Diagnostic guidelines
The child's spelling performance should be significantly below the level
expected on the basis of his or her age, general intelligence, and school
placement, and is best assessed by means of an individually administered, standardized test of spelling. The child's reading skills (with
respect to both accuracy and comprehension) should be within the normal range and there should be no history of previous significant reading
difficulties. The difficulties in spelling should not be mainly due to
grossly inadequate teaching or to the direct effects of deficits of visual,
hearing, or neurological function, and should not have been acquired as
a result of any neurological, psychiatric, or other disorder.

Although it is known that a 'pure' spelling disorder differs from reading disorders associated with spelling difficulties, little is known of the
antecedents, course, correlates, or outcome of specific spelling disorders.

Includes: specific spelling retardation (without reading disorder)

Excludes: acquired spelling disorder (R48.8)
spelling difficulties associated with a reading disorder
(F81.0)
spelling difficulties mainly attributable to inadequate teach
ing (Z55.8)

F81.2   *Specific disorder of arithmetical skills*

This disorder involves a specific impairment in arithmetical skills, which is not solely explicable on the basis of general mental retardation or of grossly inadequate schooling. The deficit concerns mastery of basic computational skills of addition, subtraction, multiplication, and division (rather than of the more abstract mathematical skills involved in algebra, trigonometry, geometry, or calculus).

Diagnostic guidelines

The child's arithmetical performance should be significantly below the level expected on the basis of his or her age, general intelligence, and school placement, and is best assessed by means of an individually administered, standardized test of arithmetic. Reading and spelling skills should be within the normal range expected for the child's mental age, preferably as assessed on individually administered, appropriately standardized tests. The difficulties in arithmetic should not be mainly due to grossly inadequate teaching, or to the direct effects of defects of visual, hearing, or neurological function, and should not have been acquired as a result of any neurological, psychiatric, or other disorder.

Arithmetical disorders have been studied less than reading disorders, and knowledge of antecedents, course, correlates, and outcome is quite limited. However, it seems that children with these disorders tend to have auditory–perceptual and verbal skills within the normal range, but impaired visuo-spatial and visual–perceptual skills; this is in contrast to many children with reading disorders. Some children have associated socio-emotional–behavioural problems but little is known about their characteristics or frequency. It has been suggested that difficulties in social interactions may be particularly common.

The arithmetical difficulties that occur are various but may include: failure to understand the concepts underlying particular arithmetical operations; lack of understanding of mathematical terms or signs; failure to recognize numerical symbols; difficulty in carrying out standard arithmetical manipulations; difficulty in understanding which numbers are relevant to the arithmetical problem being considered; difficulty in properly aligning numbers or in inserting decimal points or symbols during calculations; poor spatial organization of arithmetical calculations; and inability to learn multiplication tables satisfactorily.

Includes: developmental acalculia
               developmental arithmetical disorder
               developmental Gerstmann syndrome

Excludes: acquired arithmetical disorder (acalculia) (R48.8)
arithmetical difficulties associated with a reading or spelling
disorder (F81.1)
arithmetical difficulties mainly attributable to inadequate
teaching (Z55.8)

F81.3   ***Mixed disorder of scholastic skills***
This is an ill-defined, inadequately conceptualized (but necessary) residual category of disorders in which both arithmetical and reading or
spelling skills are significantly impaired, but in which the disorder is not
solely explicable in terms of general mental retardation or inadequate
schooling. It should be used for disorders meeting the criteria for F81.2
and either F81.0 or F81.1.

Excludes: specific disorder of arithmetical skills (F81.2)
specific reading disorder (F81.0)
specific spelling disorder (F81.1)

F81.8   ***Other developmental disorders of scholastic skills***
Includes: developmental expressive writing disorder

F81.9   ***Developmental disorder of scholastic skills, unspecified***
This category should be avoided as far as possible and should be used
only for unspecified disorders in which there is a significant disability of
learning that cannot be solely accounted for by mental retardation, visual acuity problems, or inadequate schooling.

Includes: knowledge acquisition disability NOS
learning disability NOS
learning disorder NOS

F82   **Specific developmental disorder of motor function**

The main feature of this disorder is a serious impairment in the development of motor coordination that is not solely explicable in terms of general intellectual retardation or of any specific congenital or acquired
neurological disorder (other than the one that may be implicit in the
coordination abnormality). It is usual for the motor clumsiness to be
associated with some degree of impaired performance on visuo-spatial
cognitive tasks.

Diagnostic guidelines

The child's motor coordination, on fine or gross motor tasks, should be significantly below the level expected on the basis of his or her age and general intelligence. This is best assessed on the basis of an individually administered, standardized test of fine and gross motor coordination. The difficulties in co-ordination should have been present since early in development (i.e. they should not constitute an acquired deficit), and they should not be a direct result of any defects of vision or hearing or of any diagnosable neurological disorder.

The extent to which the disorder mainly involves fine or gross motor coordination varies, and the particular pattern of motor disabilities varies with age. Developmental motor milestones may be delayed and there may be some associated speech difficulties (especially involving articulation). The young child may be awkward in general gait, being slow to learn to run, hop, and go up and down stairs. There is likely to be difficulty learning to tie shoe laces, to fasten and unfasten buttons, and to throw and catch balls. The child may be generally clumsy in fine and/or gross movements - tending to drop things, to stumble, to bump into obstacles, and to have poor handwriting. Drawing skills are usually poor, and children with this disorder are often poor at jigsaw puzzles, using constructional toys, building models, ball games, and drawing and understanding maps.

In most cases a careful clinical examination shows marked neurodevelopmental immaturities such as choreiform movements of unsupported limbs, or mirror movements and other associated motor features, as well as signs of poor fine and gross motor coordination (generally described as 'soft' neurological signs because of their normal occurrence in younger children and their lack of localizing value). Tendon reflexes may be increased or decreased bilaterally but will not be asymmetrical.

Scholastic difficulties occur in some children and may occasionally be severe; in some cases there are associated socio-emotional–behavioural problems, but little is known of their frequency or characteristics.

There is no diagnosable neurological disorder (such as cerebral palsy or muscular dystrophy). In some cases, however, there is a history of perinatal complications, such as very low birth weight or markedly premature birth.

The clumsy child syndrome has often been diagnosed as 'minimal brain dysfunction', but this term is not recommended as it has so many different and contradictory meanings.

Includes: clumsy child syndrome
              developmental coordination disorder
              developmental dyspraxia

Excludes: abnormalities of gait and mobility (R26.–)
            lack of coordination (R27.–) secondary to either mental retar
            dation (F70–F79) or some specific diagnosable neurologi
            cal disorder (G00–G99)

F83   Mixed specific developmental disorders

This is an ill-defined, inadequately conceptualized (but necessary) residual category of disorders in which there is some admixture of specific
developmental disorders of speech and language, of scholastic skills,
and/or of motor function, but in which none predominates sufficiently to
constitute the prime diagnosis. It is common for each of these specific
developmental disorders to be associated with some degree of general
impairment of cognitive functions, and this mixed category should be
used only when there is a major overlap. Thus, the category should be
used when there are dysfunctions meeting the criteria for two or more of
F80.–, F81.–, and F82.

F88[2]   Other disorders of psychological development

Includes: developmental agnosia

F89   Unspecified disorder of psychological development

Includes: developmental disorder NOS

---

[2]   F84, Pervasive developmental disorders, is included in Axis One, as explained in the
     Introduction to this book.

Axis Three
Intellectual Level

XX **Intellectual level within the normal range**

F70–F79 **Mental retardation**

Overview of this block

F70	Mild mental retardation
F71	Moderate mental retardation
F72	Severe mental retardation
F73	Profound mental retardation
F78	Other mental retardation
F79	Unspecified mental retardation

A fourth character may be used to specify the extent of associated behavioural impairment:

F7x.0	No, or minimal, impairment of behaviour
F7x.1	Significant impairment of behaviour requiring attention or treatment
F7x.8	Other impairments of behaviour
F7x.9	Without mention of impairment of behaviour

Introduction

Mental retardation is a condition of arrested or incomplete development of the mind, which is especially characterized by impairment of skills manifested during the developmental period, which contribute to the overall level of intelligence, i.e. cognitive, language, motor, and social abilities. Retardation can occur with or without any other mental or physical disorder. However, mentally retarded individuals can experience the full range of mental disorders, and the prevalence of other mental disorders is at least three to four times greater in this population than in the general population. In addition, mentally retarded individuals are at greater risk of exploitation and physical/sexual abuse. Adaptive behaviour is always impaired, but in protected social environments where support is available this impairment may not be at all obvious in subjects with mild mental retardation.

A fourth character may be used to specify the extent of the behavioural impairment, if this is not due to an associated disorder:

F7x.0   No, or minimal, impairment of behaviour
F7x.1   Significant impairment of behaviour requiring attention or treatment
F7x.8   Other impairments of behaviour
F7x.9   Without mention of impairment of behaviour

If the cause of the mental retardation is known, an additional code from ICD–10 should be used (e.g. F72 severe mental retardation plus E00.– (congenital iodine-deficiency syndrome)).

The presence of mental retardation does not rule out additional diagnoses coded elsewhere in this book. However, communication difficulties are likely to make it necessary to rely more than usual for the diagnosis upon objectively observable symptoms such as, in the case of a depressive episode, psychomotor retardation, loss of appetite and weight, and sleep disturbance.

Diagnostic guidelines

Intelligence is not a unitary characteristic but is assessed on the basis of a large number of different, more or less specific skills. Although the general tendency is for all these skills to develop to a similar level in each individual, there can be large discrepancies, especially in persons who are mentally retarded. Such people may show severe impairments in one particular area (e.g. language), or may have a particular area of higher skill (e.g. in simple visuo-spatial tasks) against a background of severe mental retardation. This presents problems when determining the diagnostic category in which a retarded person should be classified. The assessment of intellectual level should be based on whatever information is available, including clinical findings, adaptive behaviour (judged in relation to the individual's cultural background), and psychometric test performance.

For a definite diagnosis, there should be a reduced level of intellectual functioning resulting in diminished ability to adapt to the daily demands of the normal social environment. Associated mental or physical disorders have a major influence on the clinical picture and the use made of any skills. The diagnostic category chosen should therefore be based on global assessments of ability and not on any single area of specific impairment or skill. The IQ levels given are provided as a guide and should not be applied rigidly in view of the problems of cross-cultural validity. The categories given below are arbitrary divisions of a complex continuum, and cannot be defined with absolute precision. The IQ should be determined from standardized, individually administered intelligence tests for which local cultural norms have been determined, and the test selected should be appropriate to the individual's level of functioning and additional specific handicapping conditions, e.g. expressive language problems, hearing impairment, physical involvement. Scales of social maturity and adaptation, again locally standardized, should be completed if at all possible by interviewing a parent or care-provider who is familiar with the individual's skills in everyday life. Without the use of standardized procedures, the diagnosis must be regarded as a provisional estimate only.

F70   Mild mental retardation

Mildly retarded people acquire language with some delay but most achieve the ability to use speech for everyday purposes, to hold conversations, and to engage in the clinical interview. Most of them also achieve full independence in self-care (eating, washing, dressing, bowel and bladder control) and in practical and domestic skills, even if the rate of development is considerably slower than normal. The main difficulties are usually seen in academic school work, and many have particular problems in reading and writing. However, mildly retarded people can be greatly helped by education designed to develop their skills and compensate for their handicaps. Most of those in the higher ranges of mild mental retardation are potentially capable of work demanding practical rather than academic abilities, including unskilled or semiskilled manual labour. In a sociocultural context requiring little academic achievement, some degree of mild retardation may not itself represent a problem. However, if there is also noticeable emotional and social immaturity, the consequences of the handicap, e.g. inability to cope with the demands of marriage or child-rearing, or difficulty fitting in with cultural traditions and expectations, will be apparent.

In general, the behavioural, emotional, and social difficulties of the mildly mentally retarded, and the needs for treatment and support arising from them, are more closely akin to those found in people of normal intelligence than to the specific problems of the moderately and severely retarded. An organic etiology is being identified in increasing proportions of patients, although not yet in the majority.

Diagnostic guidelines
If the proper standardized IQ tests are used, the range 50 to 69 is indicative of mild retardation. Understanding and use of language tend to be

delayed to a varying degree, and executive speech problems that interfere with the development of independence may persist into adult life.
An organic etiology is identifiable in only a minority of subjects.
Associated conditions such as autism, other developmental disorders,
epilepsy, conduct disorders, or physical disability are found in varying
proportions. If such disorders are present, they should be coded independently.

Includes: feeble-mindedness
                    mild mental subnormality
                    mild oligophrenia
                    moron

F71   Moderate mental retardation

Individuals in this category are slow in developing comprehension and
use of language, and their eventual achievement in this area is limited.
Achievement of self-care and motor skills is also retarded, and some
need supervision throughout life. Progress in school work is limited, but
a proportion of these individuals learn the basic skills needed for reading, writing, and counting. Educational programmes can provide opportunities for them to develop their limited potential and to acquire some
basic skills; such programmes are appropriate for slow learners with a
low ceiling of achievement. As adults, moderately retarded people are
usually able to do simple practical work, if the tasks are carefully structured and skilled supervision is provided. Completely independent living in adult life is rarely achieved. Generally, however, such people are
fully mobile and physically active and the majority show evidence of
social development in their ability to establish contact, to communicate
with others, and to engage in simple social activities.

Diagnostic guidelines
The IQ is usually in the range 35 to 49. Discrepant profiles of abilities
are common in this group, with some individuals achieving higher levels
in visuo-spatial skills than in tasks dependent on language, while others
are markedly clumsy but enjoy social interaction and simple conversation. The level of development of language is variable: some of those
affected can take part in simple conversations while others have only
enough language to communicate their basic needs. Some never learn to
use language, though they may understand simple instructions and may
learn to use manual signs to compensate to some extent for their speech

disabilities. An organic etiology can be identified in the majority of moderately mentally retarded people. Childhood autism or other pervasive developmental disorders are present in a substantial minority, and have a major effect upon the clinical picture and the type of management needed. Epilepsy and neurological and physical disabilities are also common, although most moderately retarded people are able to walk without assistance. It is sometimes possible to identify other psychiatric conditions, but the limited level of language development may make diagnosis difficult and dependent upon information obtained from others who are familiar with the individual. Any such associated disorders should be coded independently.

Includes: imbecility
moderate mental subnormality
moderate oligophrenia

F72   Severe mental retardation

This category is broadly similar to that of moderate mental retardation in terms of the clinical picture, the presence of an organic etiology, and the associated conditions. The lower levels of achievement mentioned under F71 are also the most common in this group. Most people in this category suffer from a marked degree of motor impairment or other associated deficits, indicating the presence of clinically significant damage to or maldevelopment of the central nervous system.

Diagnostic guidelines
The IQ is usually in the range of 20 to 34.

Includes: severe mental subnormality
severe oligophrenia

F73   Profound mental retardation

The IQ in this category is estimated to be under 20, which means in practice that affected individuals are severely limited in their ability to understand or comply with requests or instructions. Most such individuals are immobile or severely restricted in mobility, incontinent, and capable at most of only very rudimentary forms of nonverbal communication. They possess little or no ability to care for their own basic needs, and require constant help and supervision.

Diagnostic guidelines
The IQ is under 20. Comprehension and use of language is limited to, at best, understanding basic commands and making simple requests. The most basic and simple visuo-spatial skills of sorting and matching may be acquired, and the affected person may be able with appropriate supervision and guidance to take a small part in domestic and practical tasks. An organic etiology can be identified in most cases. Severe neurological or other physical disabilities affecting mobility are common, as are epilepsy and visual and hearing impairments. Pervasive developmental disorders in their most severe form, especially atypical autism, are particularly frequent, especially in those who are mobile.

Includes: idiocy
profound mental subnormality
profound oligophrenia

F78   Other mental retardation

This category should be used only when assessment of the degree of intellectual retardation by means of the usual procedures is rendered particularly difficult or impossible by associated sensory or physical impairments, as in blind, deaf-mute, and severely behaviourally disturbed or physically disabled people.

F79   Unspecified mental retardation

There is evidence of mental retardation, but insufficient information is available to assign the patient to one of the above categories.

Includes: mental deficiency NOS
mental subnormality NOS
oligophrenia NOS

Axis Four

Medical Conditions from ICD-10 often associated with Mental and Behavioural Disorders

This axis contains a list of conditions in other chapters of ICD-10 that are often found in association with the disorders in Chapter V(F) itself. They are provided here so that psychiatrists recording diagnoses by means of the Clinical Descriptions and Diagnostic Guidelines have immediately to hand the ICD terms and codes that cover the associated diagnoses most likely to be encountered in ordinary clinical practice. The majority of the conditions covered are given only at the three-character level, but four-character codes are given for a selection of those diagnoses that are likely to be used most frequently. A dash following a three character code (e.g. A80.–) indicates that the full ICD-10 includes categories at the four character level but that these are not included in this abbreviated list. This dash is not inserted where at least one four character rubric has been included under the respective three digit one, even if not all the four character ones are cited. Those wishing to use the four character code where only three are cited in this list, will need to consult the full ICD-10.

As with the first three axes, a coding of XX should be given when there is no significant medical condition.

Chapter I
Certain infectious and parasitic diseases (A00–B99)

A50 *Congenital syphilis*
   A50.0   Early congenital syphilis, symptomatic
   A50.1   Early congenital syphilis, latent
   A50.2   Early congenital syphilis, unspecified
   A50.3   Late congenital syphilitic oculopathy
   A50.4   Late congenital neurosyphilis [juvenile neurosyphilis]
   A50.5   Other late congenital syphilis, symptomatic
   A50.6   Late congenital syphilis, latent
   A50.7   Late congenital syphilis, unspecified
   A50.9   Congenital syphilis, unspecified

A80.– *Acute poliomyelitis*

A81   *Slow virus infections of central nervous system*
        A81.1   Subacute sclerosing panencephalitis
        A81.2   Progressive multifocal leukoencephalopathy

B20.–   *Human immunodeficiency virus [HIV] disease resulting in infectious and parasitic diseases*

B21.–   *Human immunodeficiency virus [HIV] disease resulting in malignant neoplasms*

B22   *Human immunodeficiency virus (HIV) disease resulting in other specified diseases*
        B22.0   HIV disease resulting in encephalopathy

        Includes: HIV dementia

B23.–   *Human immunodeficiency virus [HIV] disease resulting in other conditions*

B24   *Unspecified human immunodeficiency virus [HIV] disease*

B90.–   *Sequelae of tuberculosis*

B91   *Sequelae of poliomyelitis*

B92   *Sequelae of leprosy*

B94.–   *Sequelae of other and unspecified infectious and parasitic diseases*

        Chapter II
        Neoplasms (C00–D48)

C70.–   *Malignant neoplasm of meninges*

C71.–   *Malignant neoplasm of brain*

C72.–   *Malignant neoplasm of spinal cord, cranial nerves and other parts of central nervous system*

D33.–   *Benign neoplasm of brain and other parts of central nervous system*

D42.–   *Neoplasm of uncertain and unknown behaviour of meninges*

D43.–   *Neoplasm of uncertain and unknown behaviour of brain and central nervous system*

Chapter IV
Endocrine, nutritional and metabolic diseases (E00–E90)

E00.–   *Congenital iodine–deficiency syndrome*

E01.–   *Iodine-deficiency-related thyroid disorders and allied conditions*

E02   *Subclinical iodine-deficiency hypothyroidism*

E03   *Other hypothyroidism*

E03.2 *Hypothyroidism due to medicaments and other exogenous substances*

E05.–   *Thyrotoxicosis [hyperthyroidism]*

E10   *Insulin-dependent diabetes mellitus*
      Includes: diabetes (mellitus):
               brittle
               juvenile-onset
               ketosis-prone
               type I
      E10.0   Insulin-dependent diabetes mellitus with coma
      Includes: Diabetic:
               coma with or without ketoacidosis
               hyperosmolar coma
               hypoglycaemic coma
               Hyperglycaemic coma NOS
      E10.1   Insulin-dependent diabetes mellitus with ketoacidosis
      Includes: Diabetic without mention of coma:
               acidosis
               ketoacidosis

E15   *Nondiabetic hypoglycaemic coma*

E22   **Hyperfunction of pituitary gland**
          E22.0   Acromegaly and pituitary gigantism
          E22.1   Hyperprolactinaemia

          Includes: drug-induced hyperprolactinaemia

E23.–   *Hypofunction and other disorders of pituitary gland*

E24.–   *Cushing's syndrome*

E30   **Disorders of puberty, not elsewhere classified**
          E30.0   Delayed puberty
          E30.1   Precocious puberty

E34   **Other endocrine disorders**
          E34.3   Short stature, not elsewhere classified

E51   **Thiamine deficiency**
          E51.2   Wernicke's encephalopathy

E64.–   *Sequel of malnutrition and other nutritional deficiencies*

E66.–   *Obesity*

E70   **Disorders of aromatic amino-acid metabolism**
          E70.0   Classical phenylketonuria

E71   **Disorders of branched-chain amino-acid metabolism and fatty-acid metabolism**
          E71.0   Maple-syrup-urine disease

E74.–   *Other disorders of carbohydrate metabolism*

E80.–   *Disorders of porphyrin and bilirubin metabolism*

Chapter VI
Diseases of the nervous system (G00–G99)

G00.–   *Bacterial meningitis, not elsewhere classified*

Includes: haemophilus, pneumococcal, streptococcal, staphylococcal and other bacterial meningitis

G02.–   ***Meningitis in other infectious and parasitic diseases classified elsewhere***

G03.–   ***Meningitis due to other and unspecified causes***

G04.–   ***Encephalitis, myelitis and encephalomyelitis***

G06   ***Intracranial and intraspinal abscess and granuloma***
            G06.2   Extradural and subdural abscess, unspecified

G09   ***Sequelae of inflammatory diseases of central nervous system***

G10   ***Huntington's disease***

G11.–   ***Hereditary ataxia***

G20   ***Parkinson's disease***

G21   ***Secondary parkinsonism***
            G21.0   Malignant neuroleptic syndrome
            G21.1   Other drug-induced secondary parkinsonism
            G21.2   Secondary parkinsonism due to other external agents
            G21.3   Postencephalitic parkinsonism

G24   ***Dystonia***
            Includes: dyskinesia

            G24.0   Drug-induced dystonia
            G24.3   Spasmodic torticollis
            G24.8   Other dystonia

            Includes: tardive dyskinesia

G25.–   ***Other extrapyramidal and movement disorders***
            Includes: restless legs syndrome, drug-induced tremor, myoclonus, chorea, tics

G32.–   ***Other degenerative disorders of nervous system in diseases classified elsewhere***

G35   *Multiple sclerosis*

G37   *Other demyelinating diseases of central nervous system*
G37.0   Diffuse sclerosis

Includes: periaxial encephalitis; Schilder's disease

G40   *Epilepsy*
G40.0   Localization-related (focal) (partial) idiopathic epilepsy and epileptic syndromes with seizures of localized onset

Includes: benign childhood epilepsy with centrotemporal EEG spikes or occipital EEG paroxysms

G40.1   Localization-related (focal) (partial) symptomatic epilepsy and epileptic syndromes with simple partial seizures

Includes: attacks without alteration of consciousness

G40.2   Localization-related (focal) (partial) symptomatic epilepsy and epileptic syndromes with complex partial seizures

Includes: attacks with alteration of consciousness, often with automatisms

G40.3   Generalized idiopathic epilepsy and epileptic syndromes
G40.4   Other generalized epilepsy and epileptic syndromes

Includes: salaam attacks

G40.5   Special epileptic syndromes

Includes: epileptic seizures related to alcohol, drugs and sleep deprivation

G40.6   Grand mal seizures, unspecified (with or without petit mal)
G40.7   Petit mal, unspecified, without grand mal seizures

G41.–   *Status epilepticus*

G43.–   *Migraine*

G44.–   *Other headache syndromes*

G45.–   *Transient cerebral ischaemic attacks and related syndromes*

G47   *Sleep disorders*
G47.2   Disorders of the sleep–wake schedule
G47.4   Narcolepsy and cataplexy

G70   *Myasthenia gravis and other myoneural disorders*
G70.0   Myasthenia gravis

G80.–   *Infantile cerebral palsy*
Includes: Little's disease
Excludes: hereditary spastic paraplegia (G11.4)

G83.–   *Other paralytic syndromes*

G91.–   *Hydrocephalus*

G92   *Toxic encephalopathy*

G93   *Other disorders of brain*
G93.1   Anoxic brain damage, not elsewhere classified
G93.3   Postviral fatigue syndrome

Includes: benign myalgic encephalomyelitis

G93.4   Encephalopathy, unspecified

G97   *Postprocedural disorders of nervous system, not elsewhere classified*
G97.0   Cerebrospinal fluid leak from spinal puncture

Chapter VII
Diseases of the eye and adnexa (H00–H59)

H40   *Glaucoma*
H40.6   Glaucoma secondary to drugs

H53.–   *Visual disturbances*

H54   *Blindness and low vision*
H54.2   Low vision, both eyes
H54.5   Low vision, one eye

Four

Chapter VIII
Diseases of the ear and mastoid process (H60–H95)

H90.–   *Conductive and sensorineural hearing loss*

H91.–   *Other hearing loss*

Chapter IX
Diseases of the circulatory system (I00–I99)

I60.–   *Subarachnoid haemorrhage*

I61.–   *Intracerebral haemorrhage*

I62   *Other nontraumatic intracranial haemorrhage*
           I62.0   Subdural haemorrhage (acute) (nontraumatic)
           I62.1   Nontraumatic extradural haemorrhage

I63.–   *Cerebral infarction*

I64   *Stroke, not specified as haemorrhage or infarction*

I65.–   *Occlusion and stenosis of precerebral arteries, not resulting in cerebral infarction*

I66.–   *Occlusion and stenosis of cerebral arteries, not resulting in cerebral infarction*

I67   *Other cerebrovascular diseases*
           I67.2   Cerebral atherosclerosis
           I67.3   Progressive vascular leukoencephalopathy

           Includes: Binswanger's disease

           I67.4   Hypertensive encephalopathy

I69.–   *Sequel of cerebrovascular disease*

I95   *Hypotension*
           I95.2   Hypotension due to drugs

Chapter X
Diseases of the respiratory system (J00–J99)

J10   *Influenza due to identified influenza virus*
        J10.8   Influenza with other manifestations, influenza virus identified

J11   *Influenza, virus not identified*
        J11.8   Influenza with other manifestations, virus not identified

J45.– *Asthma*

Chapter XI
Diseases of the digestive system (K00–K93)

K25.– *Gastric ulcer*

K26.– *Duodenal ulcer*

K27.– *Peptic ulcer, site unspecified*

K29   *Gastritis and duodenitis*

K30   *Dyspepsia*

K51.– *Ulcerative colitis*

K58.– *Irritable bowel syndrome*

K59.– *Other functional intestinal disorders*

K70.– *Alcoholic liver disease*

K71.– *Toxic liver disease*
        Includes: drug-induced liver disease

K86   *Other diseases of pancreas*

Four

Chapter XII
Diseases of the skin and subcutaneous tissue (L00–L99)

L20.–   *Atopic dermatitis*

L21.–   *Seborrhoeic dermatitis*

L22   *Diaper [napkin] dermatitis*

L23.–   *Allergic contact dermatitis*

L24.–   *Irritant contact dermatitis*

L25.–   *Unspecified contact dermatitis*

L26   *Exfoliative dermatitis*

L27.–   *Dermatitis due to substances taken internally*

L28.–   *Lichen simplex chronicus and prurigo*

L29.–   *Pruritus*
           Excludes: psychogenic pruritus (F45.8 to be coded in Axis One)

L30.–   *Other dermatitis*

L40.–   *Psoriasis*

L98   *Other disorders of skin and subcutaneous tissue, not elsewhere classi-*
           fied
           L98.1   Factitial dermatitis
           Includes: neurotic excoriation

Chapter XIII
Diseases of the musculoskeletal system and connective tissue
(M00–M99)

M32.–   *Systemic lupus erythematosus*
           M32.0   Drug-induced systemic lupus erythematosus

M54.–   *Dorsalgia*

Chapter XIV
Diseases of the genitourinary system (N00–N99)

N47   *Redundant prepuce, phimosis and paraphimosis*

N91.–   *Absent, scanty and rare menstruation*

N94   *Pain and other conditions associated with female genital organs and menstrual cycle*
N94.3   Premenstrual tension syndrome
N94.4   Primary dysmenorrhoea
N94.5   Secondary dysmenorrhoea
N94.6   Dysmenorrhoea, unspecified

Chapter XV
Pregnancy, childbirth and the puerperium (O00–O99)

O04.–   *Medical abortion*

O05.–   *Other abortion*

O07.–   *Failed attempted abortion*

O35   *Maternal care for known or suspected fetal abnormality and damage*
O35.4   Maternal care for (suspected) damage to fetus from alcohol
O35.5   Maternal care for (suspected) damage to fetus by drugs

O99   *Other maternal diseases classifiable elsewhere but complicating pregnancy, childbirth and puerperium*
O99.3   Mental disorders and diseases of the nervous system complicating pregnancy, childbirth and the puerperium

Includes: conditions in F00–F99 and G00–G99

Chapter XVI
Certain conditions originating in the perinatal period (P00-P96)

P35.-   *Congenital viral diseases (including congenital rubella syndrome)*

P96   *Other conditions originating in the perinatal period*

P96.1   Neonatal withdrawal symptoms from maternal use of drugs of addiction

Chapter XVII
Congenital malformations, deformations, and chromosomal abnormalities (Q00–Q99)

Q02   *Microcephaly*

Q03.–   *Congenital hydrocephalus*

Q04.–   *Other congenital malformations of brain*

Q05.–   *Spina bifida*

Q52.–   *Other congenital malformations of female genitalia*

Q53.–   *Undescended testicle*

Q54.–   *Hypospadias*

Q55.–   *Other congenital malformations of male genital organs*

Q56.–   *Indeterminate sex and pseudohermaphroditism*

Q75.–   *Other congenital malformations of skull and face bones*

Q85   *Phakomatoses, not elsewhere classified*
           Q85.0   Neurofibromatosis (nonmalignant)
           Q85.1   Tuberous sclerosis

Q86   *Congenital malformation syndromes due to known exogenous causes, not elsewhere classified*
           Q86.0   Fetal alcohol syndrome (dysmorphic)

Q90   *Down's syndrome*
           Q90.0   Trisomy 21, meiotic nondisjunction
           Q90.1   Trisomy 21, mosaicism (mitotic nondisjunction)
           Q90.2   Trisomy 21, translocation
           Q90.9   Down's syndrome, unspecified

Q91.– *Edwards' syndrome and Patau's syndrome*

Q93 *Monosomies and deletions from the autosomes, not elsewhere classified*
Q93.4 Deletion of short arm of chromosome 5

Includes: *cri-du-chat* syndrome

Q96.– *Turner's syndrome*

Q97.– *Other sex chromosome abnormalities, female phenotype, not elsewhere classified*

Q98 *Other sex chromosome abnormalities, male phenotype, not elsewhere classified*
Q98.0 Klinefelter's syndrome karyotype 47, XXY
Q98.1 Klinefelter's syndrome, male with more than two X chromosomes
Q98.2 Klinefelter's syndrome, male with 46, XX karyotype
Q98.4 Klinefelter's syndrome, unspecified

Q99.– *Other chromosome abnormalities, not elsewhere classified*

Chapter XVIII
Symptoms, signs and abnormal clinical and laboratory findings, not elsewhere classified (R00–R99)

R55 *Syncope and collapse*

R56 *Convulsions, not elsewhere classified*
R56.0 Febrile convulsions
R56.8 Other and unspecified convulsions

R62 *Lack of expected normal physiological development*
R62.0 Delayed milestone
R62.8 Other lack of expected normal physiological development
R62.9 Lack of expected normal physiological development, unspecified

R63 *Symptoms and signs concerning food and fluid intake*
R63.0 Anorexia

Four

R63.4   Abnormal weight loss
R63.5   Abnormal weight gain

R78.–   ***Findings of drugs and other substances, normally not found in blood***
Includes: alcohol (R78.0); opiate drug (R78.1); cocaine (R78.2); hallucinogen (R78.3); other drugs of addictive potential (R78.4); psychotropic drug (R.78.5); abnormal level of lithium (R78.8)

R83   ***Abnormal findings in cerebrospinal fluid***

R90.–   ***Abnormal findings on diagnostic imaging of central nervous system***

R94   ***Abnormal results of function studies***
R94.0   Abnormal results of function studies of central nervous system

Includes: abnormal electroencephalogram [EEG]

Chapter XIX
Injury, poisoning and certain other consequences of external causes
(S00–T98)

S04.–   ***Injury of cranial nerves***

S06   ***Intracranial injury***
S06.0   Concussion
S06.1   Traumatic cerebral oedema
S06.2   Diffuse brain injury
S06.3   Focal brain injury
S06.4   Epidural haemorrhage
S06.5   Traumatic subdural haemorrhage
S06.6   Traumatic subarachnoid haemorrhage
S06.7   Intracranial injury with prolonged coma
S06.8   Other intracranial injuries

T36.– – T50.– ***Poisoning by drugs, medicaments and biological substances***
Includes: overdosage of these substances
wrong substances given or taken in error

T52.–   ***Toxic effects of organic solvents***

T74.–   *Maltreatment syndromes*

T90.–   *Sequelae of injuries to head*

Chapter XX
External causes of morbidity and mortality (V0I–Y98)

Intentional self-harm (X60–X84)
Includes: purposely self-inflicted poisoning or injury; suicide

X60   *Intentional self-poisoning by and exposure to nonopioid analgesics,*
antipyretics and antirheumatics

X61   *Intentional self-poisoning by and exposure to antiepileptic, sedative-*
hypnotic, antiparkinsonism and psychotropic drugs, not elsewhere
classified
Includes: antidepressants, barbiturates, neuroleptics, psychostimulants

X62   *Intentional self-poisoning by and exposure to narcotics and psy-*
chodysleptics [hallucinogens], not elsewhere classified
Includes: cannabis (derivatives), cocaine, codeine, heroin, lysergide
          [LSD], mescaline, methadone, morphine, opium (alkaloids)

X63   *Intentional self-poisoning by and exposure to other drugs acting on*
the autonomic nervous systems

X64   *Intentional self-poisoning by and exposure to other and unspecified*
drugs and biological substances

X65   *Intentional self-poisoning by and exposure to alcohol*

X66   *Intentional self-poisoning by and exposure to organic solvents and*
halogenated hydrocarbons and their vapours

X67   *Intentional self-poisoning by and exposure to other gases and vapours*
Includes: carbon monoxide; utility gas

X68   *Intentional self-poisoning by and exposure to pesticides*

X69   ***Intentional self-poisoning by and exposure to other and unspecified chemicals and noxious substances***
Includes: corrosive aromatics, acids and caustic alkalis

X70   ***Intentional self-harm by hanging, strangulation and suffocation***

X71   ***Intentional self-harm by drowning and submersion***

X72   ***Intentional self-harm by handgun discharge***

X73   ***Intentional self-harm by rifle, shotgun and larger firearm discharge***

X74   ***Intentional self-harm by other and unspecified firearm discharge***

X75   ***Intentional self-harm by explosive material***

X76   ***Intentional self-harm by fire and flames***

X77   ***Intentional self-harm by steam, hot vapours and hot objects***

X78   ***Intentional self-harm by sharp object***

X79   ***Intentional self-harm by blunt object***

X80   ***Intentional self-harm by jumping from a high place***

X81   ***Intentional self-harm by jumping or lying before moving object***

X82   ***Intentional self-harm by crashing of motor vehicle***

X83   ***Intentional self-harm by other specified means***
Includes: electrocution, caustic substances (except poisoning)

X84   ***Intentional self-harm by unspecified means***

Assault (X85–Y09)

These codings should however normally be made in Axis Five under 6.4 Sexual abuse or 6.5 Personal frightening experiences

Drugs, medicaments and biological substances causing adverse effects in therapeutic use (Y40–Y59)

Sequelae of external causes of morbidity and mortality (Y85-Y89)

Note: Categories Y85-Y89 are to be used to indicate circumstances as the cause of death, impairment or disability from sequelae or 'late effects', which are themselves classified elsewhere. The sequelae include conditions reported as such, or occurring as 'late effects' one year or more after the originating event.

Y85   *Sequelae of transport accidents*

Y86   *Sequelae of other accidents*

Y87   *Sequelae of intentional self-harm, assault and events of undetermined intent*

Y89   *Sequelae of other external causes*

Y46   *Antiepileptics and antiparkinsonism drugs*

Y47.–   *Sedatives, hypnotics and antianxiety drugs*

Y49   *Psychotropic drugs, not elsewhere classified*
      Y49.0   Tricyclic and tetracyclic antidepressants
      Y49.1   Monoamine-oxidase-inhibitor antidepressants
      Y49.2   Other and unspecified antidepressants
      Y49.3   Phenothiazine antipsychotics and neuroleptics
      Y49.4   Butyrophenone and thioxanthene neuroleptics
      Y49.5   Other antipsychotics and neuroleptics
      Y49.6   Psychodysleptics [hallucinogens]
      Y49.7   Psychostimulants with abuse potential
      Y49.8   Other psychotropic drugs, not elsewhere classified
      Y49.9   Psychotropic drug, unspecified

Y50.–   *Central nervous system stimulants, not elsewhere classified*

Y51.–   *Drugs primarily affecting the autonomic nervous system*

Y57.–   *Other and unspecified drugs and medicaments*

Four

Axis Five — Associated Abnormal Psychosocial Situations

List of categories

00 No significant distortion or inadequacy of the psychosocial environment

1 Abnormal intrafamilial relationships
    1.0   Lack of warmth in parent–child relationships (Z62.4)[1]
    1.1   Intrafamilial discord among adults (Z63.8)
    1.2   Hostility towards or scapegoating of the child (Z62.3)
    1.3   Physical child abuse (Z61.6)
    1.4   Sexual abuse (within the family) (Z61.4)
    1.8   Other

2 Mental disorder, deviance or handicap in the child's primary support group (Z58.8 + Z63.8)
    2.0   Parental mental disorder/deviance
    2.1   Parental handicap/disability
    2.2   Disability in sibling
    2.8   Other

3 Inadequate or distorted intrafamilial communication (Z63.8)

4 Abnormal qualities of upbringing
    4.0   Parental overprotection (Z62.1)
    4.1   Inadequate parental supervision/control (Z62.0)
    4.2   Experiential privation (Z62.5)
    4.3   Inappropriate parental pressures (Z62.6)
    4.8   Other (Z62.8)

5 Abnormal immediate environment
    5.0   Institutional upbringing (Z62.2)
    5.1   Anomalous parenting situation (Z80.1)
    5.2   Isolated family (Z60.8)
    5.3   Living conditions that create a potentially hazardous psychosocial situation (Z59.1)
    5.8   Other (Z60.8)

Five

---

[1] These Z codes refer to the position of these categories within Chapter XXI (Factors influencing health status and contact with health services) in the ICD-10.

6   Acute life events
    6.0   Loss of a love relationship (Z61.0)
    6.1   Removals from home carrying significant contextual threat (Z61.1)
    6.2   Negatively altered pattern of family relationships (Z61.2)
    6.3   Events resulting in loss of self esteem (Z61.3)
    6.4   Sexual abuse (extrafamilial) (Z61.5)
    6.5   Personal frightening experience (Z61.7)
    6.8   Other (Z61.8)

7   Societal stressors
    7.0   Persecution or adverse discrimination (Z60.5)
    7.1   Migration or social transplantation (Z60.3)
    7.8   Other

8   Chronic interpersonal stress associated with school/work (Z55 refers to school and Z56 to work)
    8.0   Discordant relationships with peers (Z55.4) Z56.4)
    8.1   Scapegoating of child by teachers or work supervisors (Z55.4) (Z56.4)
    8.2   Unrest in the school/work situation (Z55.8) (Z56.7)
    8.8   Other

9   Stressful events/situations resulting from the child's own disorder/disability (Z72.8) (within ICD-10 these could be coded under the same categories used where these have not resulted from the child's own disorder/disability, i.e. Z62.1, Z61.1 and Z61.3 respectively.)
    9.0   Institutional upbringing
    9.1   Removal from home carrying significant contextual threat
    9.2   Events resulting in loss of self-esteem
    9.8   Other

Introduction

This axis provides a means of coding those aspects of the child's psychosocial situation that are significantly abnormal in the context of the child's level of development, past experiences and prevailing sociocultural circumstances. The categories included on this axis have been chosen on the basis of evidence that they may constitute significant psychiatric risk factors. However, codings should be made strictly in terms of whether the child's situation fulfils the guidelines for the categories, irrespective of whether such psychosocial circumstances are considered to be a direct cause of the psychiatric disorder. This approach is necessary because in most cases there is inadequate evidence to come to a firm decision on the causal role in an individual case; because it is common for psychosocial adversities to constitute contributory etiological factors but yet not a sufficient cause for disorder; and because clinicians differ in their views on the importance of psychosocial factors as causal influences. Nevertheless, because the axis is intended to cover factors that may have influenced the genesis of disorder, or may influence the future course of the disorder, situations that are likely to have been brought about as a consequence of the patient's own actions or symptomatic behaviour should be *excluded* from codings 1 to 8 (there is provision for such events/situations resulting from the child's disorder/disability under code 9).

For each category, a rating code of '2' means that the situation definitely applied during the specified time period and was of a type and severity that definitely met the diagnostic guidelines for the category. A rating code of '1' means that the situation definitely applied during the specified time period, was of a type that fulfilled the category guidelines, but was of a severity that fell just short of the specified criteria in spite of being judged clinically abnormal and potentially significant. A rating code of '0' means that the patient's psychosocial situation (with respect to the features in that rating code) was within a broadly defined normal range (i.e. including minor abnormalities of little clinical significance). A rating code of '8' means that the situation is not applicable to that particular patient (i.e. it *could not* have occurred to the patient given his or her overall circumstances); a rating code of '9' means that there is insufficient information to make the rating.

It will be appreciated that this axis is not intended to include all types of potential etiological factors. Thus, for example, genetic factors are not encompassed unless they happen to be associated with one or other of the specified types of abnormalities of the psychosocial environment. Similarly, the axis does not provide for coverage of any stresses associated with puberty or with any other physical transitions. Rather it provides for a means of some sort of systematic coding to describe the main types of abnormal psychosocial situations that apply to the child's environmental circumstances. Even so, clinicians may consider that psychosocial factors that fail to fulfil the specified criteria have nevertheless played a role, perhaps even a crucial role, in etiology. For example, in a vulnerable child the mere starting of school or the birth of a sibling may constitute a significant stressor. Inevitably, a limited set of codings can-

Five

not cover all the many varieties of psychosocial situations that may be relevant in individual cases. Instead, the categories are confined to those in which the available evidence suggests that they carry a substantial psychiatric risk for a significant proportion of children.

The categories describe selected facets of children's environmental circumstances. It may be expected that often several categories will apply; moreover it will be common for these to overlap or reflect different aspects of what is basically the same situation. For example, parental mental disorder may be associated with family discord. However, the intention is, *not* to attempt any overall categorization of the theoretically inferred 'basic' or 'underlying' family psychopathology, but rather to categorize the several different dimensions that may have differing types of impact on the child.

Time frame

This classification provides a means of coding those abnormal psychosocial situations for which the available evidence suggests that they carry a significant psychiatric risk for a substantial proportion of children. Such situations may have been operative in infancy creating a vulnerability that long anteceded the onset of psychiatric disorder; they may have had their main effect in the months immediately preceding onset (thus acting as a precipitant of disorder); or they may be current with their main effect on course rather than onset. Clinicians and researchers will want to focus on different time periods for different purposes and the classification can be applied to any time period that may be chosen. However, in order to avoid ambiguity, and hence unreliability, it is desirable when using the classification to make explicit the chosen time period.

Codings have been expressed in terms of their reference to the whole period of the child's life. For many purposes, however, clinicians and researchers may want to code those psychosocial situations operative only during the 6 months immediately preceding the time of assessment. This period is long enough for judgements to be made on the quality of psychosocial situations (and long enough for them to have an impact on the child), but yet short enough largely to avoid major problems resulting from changes over time in children's psychosocial circumstances. Alternatively, if the focus is mainly on precipitants of disorders, it may be desirable (in addition or instead) to code those that were operative during the 6 months immediately preceding the onset of the disorder that led to psychiatric referral. A third alternative would be to code on the basis of evidence that the situation has played a role in causative processes. Users adopting this option are recommended to develop their own operational rules on how to make a causal inference. The procedure followed here is to refer to the child's whole life. This has the attraction of covering all situations likely to have impinged on the child but also the major disadvantage that there will be coding difficulties when situations have varied substantially during the child's lifetime. It is left open to users of the classification to make their own decisions on the time frame for coding.

Categorical or dimensional coding

The classification provides a means of coding 9 main types of psychosocial situations, most of which are subdivided, so that there are 40 codings in all. Each coding describes a particular aspect or feature of the child's psychosocial situation. By their nature, such aspects or features are not mutually exclusive and it is clear that in practice it is common for several, or even many, to be applicable. The classification, as presented here, does not specify whether a dimensional or categorical approach should be employed and several different formats are possible.

The most reliable and valid format is likely to be provided by a dimensional structure in which separate codings of '0', '1' or '2' (see above) are made for each and every one of the 40 specified situations. This is the recommended approach. However, the classification can equally easily be employed in a multi-category format in which raters code only those situations that apply in any individual case. This format is less easy to handle statistically, however, because of the great variations between cases and between raters in the number of situations coded. This problem may be diminished by specifying that the codings be made in order of psychiatric importance and/or that no more than a specified number of codings may be employed. Both carry the price of additional unreliability in judgement and importance, and this is not a recommended procedure.

00   No significant distortion or inadequacy of the psychosocial environment

The patient's psychosocial circumstances are within broadly defined normal limits, so that both acute stressors and chronic adversities are of a mildness thought to be of little potential clinical significance. A coding of 00 means that no other category on this axis warrants a '1' or '2' coding.

Five

1   Abnormal intrafamilial relationships

This category concerns adverse patterns of interactions and relationships within the family that are inimical to a child's social/emotional development. The adverse family relationships under this heading are known to be associated with abnormal development within a number of different societies, although the mechanisms by which the adversities have their effects are not well understood. Some of the adversities involve the child's relationships with other family members directly; others concern the overall family atmosphere within which the child is being raised.

A child may experience one, some or all of these adversities at the same time. It is anticipated that although modes of expression and thresholds for rating will vary cross-culturally, deficiencies or distortions in these areas will be identifiably similar in each culture. As a general principle in rating, the *presence* of the abnormality should be coded *regardless* of compensating positive experiences or environmental features.

By their nature, all relationships concern two-way interactions, which will be influenced by the behaviour of both participants. Accordingly, it is likely that, to a varying extent, abnormal intrafamilial relationships may have arisen in part as a result of the child's own actions, attitudes or responses. In any individual case it will often be difficult to judge how far that has been so. Codings should be made solely on the basis of the abnormality of other people's behaviour, irrespective of the child's own contribution to the poor relationship.

1.0   *Lack of warmth in parent–child relationships*

A marked lack of expressed positive feelings towards the child in the home by the child's parental figure(s). Warmth is expressed through the way in which the parent talks to the child and through nonverbal behaviours such as affectionate touching or physical comfort. The context and frequency of such overt expressions of warmth varies cross-culturally both overall and by the sex of the parent. The level of expressed warmth should be judged according to the parental behaviour that a child within that culture might normally expect to receive and to observe other children receiving. A lack of positive feelings should not be confused with the presence of critical or negative ones. It is quite possible for a warm parent to be critical of his or her child's behaviour, and this may be particularly occur when the child is currently showing problems.

Diagnostic guidelines

Lack of warmth is characteristically shown by a failure to report the child's qualities or achievements positively or with pride, and/or to discuss his/her problems or anxieties in a sympathetic or concerned manner.

The overall affective tone of the parent–child relationship constitutes the basis for rating. The specific ways in which this is shown vary from family to family but to be categorized as showing definite lack of warmth the relationship should have at least two of the following characteristics:

(a) when talking to the child the parent adopts a dismissive or insensitive tone; or

(b) interest in the child's activities, successes or accomplishments is lacking; or

(c) sympathy for the child's difficulties is not evident; or

(d) praise and encouragement is given only rarely; or

(e) anxious behaviour is met only with irritation or peremptory injunctions to behave; or

(f) physical comfort for anxiety or distress is brief, ritualized or absent (parental success in calming the child is not necessary: it is the quality of the attempt that is important).

For information on some parental figures it may be necessary to rely on reports from other members of the household. In this case only reports of behaviour should be taken into account, not generalized statements about the parent/child relationship. Such behavioural evidence would include the parent not showing any interest in the child, not asking the child about his/her interest or activities, seldom playing with him or her, not showing pleasure or pride in the child's successes or accomplishments, and/or behaving in a way consistent with the criteria for rating lack of warmth in a parent-informant. For coding of lack of warmth to be made it is necessary that the lack be (i) marked, (ii) definite, (iii) persistent over time, (iv) pervasive over situations, and (v) clearly abnormal in relation to subcultural norms. Emotional reserve or lack of enthusiasm is not sufficient for coding lack of warmth.

The lack of warmth must involve the relationship of one or both parents with the child (i.e. lack of warmth between the two parents is not relevant); however it is not necessary that the lack apply to both parents. The lack may reflect a specific abnormality in the parent-child relationship or it may stem from a more generalized parental deficit (such as

Five

with a schizophrenic defect state). The coding of lack of warmth should be made if the criteria are met irrespective of whether or not the lack derives from an abnormality noted on a different psychosocial coding (e.g. parental mental disorder).

1.1   Intrafamilial discord among adults

Intrafamilial discord concerns discord between the child's parents, or between other adult members of the child's household (including the child's siblings if they are 16 years of age or older). It does *not* include discord between the parents and the child him/herself (which is covered by category 1.2). The discord must be overt as evidenced by active negative altercations or by a persisting atmosphere of severe tension consequent upon markedly strained relationships. A lack of affection or a paucity of positive interaction is not sufficient for a coding of discord, nor are brief repeated episodes of irritability; there must be serious active negative interchange. Ordinarily, discord involves two-way negative interchanges but one-sided verbal or physical abuse should also be included.

Diagnostic guidelines

There are marked individual differences, as well as subcultural variations, in the extent to which people express their dissatisfactions, disagreements or irritation in open quarrels. Discord should be coded only when it clearly falls outside the normal range in the child's subculture. Discord should be regarded as abnormal when:

(a)   it results in severe or prolonged loss of control; or
(b)   it is associated with generalization of hostile or critical feelings; or
(c)   it is associated with a persisting atmosphere of severe interpersonal violence (hitting or striking the other person); or
(d)   leaving the home in a temper or locking the other person out of the home.

Generalization of hostile or critical feelings may be shown by:

(a)   denigration of or insults about the other person's family, friends or background; or
(b)   irrelevant reference to episodes or happenings in the past that reflect badly on the other person;
(c)   sleeping apart following a quarrel; or
(d)   prolonged periods of not speaking; or
(e)   leaving the home to sleep elsewhere following discord.

A persistent atmosphere of tension may be evident by:

(a) frequent sarcastic, dismissive or denigrating remarks about the other person; or

(b) a persisting tendency to respond to neutral or mildly negative remarks with strongly negative responses; or

(c) a persisting tendency for mildly negative interactions to escalate into prolonged coercive or hostile interchanges.

The coding should reflect the predominant situation during the specified time period. Isolated severe quarrels that were unaccompanied by a persisting atmosphere of tension would not ordinarily be sufficient for a coding of discord (but, if severe, they might be relevant for a coding under '6': acute or recurrent life events). However, discord should be coded if the altercations are severe and frequent, or if there is a persistently tense atmosphere, even if there are associated periods of harmony or positive interaction.

Discord between parents who are living apart (as between divorced parents over access to the child) is relevant for coding on this category provided that (a) the child has an ongoing relationship with both parent-figures and (b) the discord is of a type and level that meets the general criteria above. Discord between adults in the child's home who are not the child's parents is also relevant for coding. Thus, discord may apply to the relationships between a biological parent and a step-parent; between a parent and cohabiting lover; between parents and grandparents who live in the same household; between the parents and an adult child; between the parents and an adult relative or lodger sharing the same household.

1.2   Hostility towards or scapegoating of the child

This category refers to personally focused (or targeted) marked negative feelings of one or both parents (or parent surrogates or other adult members of the child's household) towards the child. Thus, it includes specific hostility towards or scapegoating of the child but it excludes general discord or negative feeling that impinges roughly equally on all members of the family. The negative feelings must be specifically directed towards the child, but it is possible for the scapegoating to apply to more than one child in the family.

Diagnostic guidelines

At its most extreme form, the parental behaviour amounts to psychological abuse in which the child is systematically tormented, humiliated and denigrated. However, the category also includes similarly focused hostile behaviour that clearly falls outside broadly defined normal limits but which falls short of a severity that might be accepted by a Court as justifying removal of the child from its parents on the basis of abuse. The coding requires that:

(i)   the negative parental behaviour towards the child is clearly abnormal in form and/or degree; and
(ii)   it is specifically focused on the child as an individual; and
(iii) it is persistent over time and pervasive over several child behaviours (i.e. an excessive parental reaction to just one or two specific child actions would not be adequate for coding).

The hostility/scapegoating may be shown by:

(a)   an unreasonable tendency automatically to blame the child for problems, or difficulties, or wrongdoing in the household; or
(b)   a general tendency to attribute the child with negative characteristics; or
(c)   criticisms of the child that extend to a general denigration of the child as a person, that generalize to past misdeeds or which include expectations of future misdeeds; or
(d)   a clear tendency specifically to 'pick on' the child or to involve the child in quarrels when the adult is feeling miserable, irritable or bad tempered;
(e)   treating the child unfairly in relation to other members of the family – with excessive workload or responsibilities, a lack of involvement in positive family interactions; or marked lack of attention to the child's needs or difficulties; or
(f)   severe punitive measures such as locking the child in confined or dark spaces such as cupboards or cellars.

1.3   Physical child abuse

Physical abuse includes any clear examples of incidents in which the child has been injured by any adult in the household to an extent that is medically significant or that involves forms of violence that are abnormal in form for the subculture.

Diagnostic guidelines

Cultures vary considerably in the extent to which it is regarded as acceptable to use corporal methods as a means of punishing children. Nevertheless, physical abuse may be considered to have occurred when:

(a)   the punishment has been sufficiently severe to result in lacerations, fractures, dislocated joints or marked bruising; or

(b)   punishment has involved hitting the child with hard or sharp implements such as sticks or belts with buckles (hitting with a slipper or a leather strap may amount to abuse but in some subcultures it need not necessarily do so if moderate in degree and well controlled); or

(c)   the punishment has involved a clear and severe loss of control, as shown by throwing the child against a wall or pushing the child downstairs; or

(d)   the violence has involved unusual and unacceptable forms of physical trauma, as shown by burning or scalding the child, tying up the child or holding the head under water.

Physical abuse may occur either as a consequence of physical punishment that has been carried to excess as a result of loss of self-control or of deliberate malicious maltreatment.

Excludes: physical abuse by someone outside the household (consider coding 6.5).

1.4   Sexual abuse (within the family)

Sexual abuse within the family includes sexual relationships that are incestuous (because they occur between family members legally prohibited from marrying) and also non-incestuous relationships between the child and other older members of the child's household in which a significant element of power or status has been used to induce the child to engage in the sexual activity. Thus, abuse would include sexual acts by biological or adoptive parents, step-parents, older siblings, other relatives in the home, lodgers or family friends.

Sexual abuse that occurs within the family or household context is included in this section because usually it involves a serious distortion of family or household relationships; nevertheless it should be coded on the basis of the sexual acts (and not on any inferences about distorted relationships).

Diagnostic guidelines

Cultures vary in the extent to which children are allowed to see their parents in the nude, in the age to which children are washed in the bath by parents, in children's sharing of the parental bed and in the age at which children are given personal privacy from their parents. However, sexual abuse may be considered to have occurred when:

(a)   there has been any genital contact between the older person and child; or

(b)   there has been any manipulation of the child's breasts or genitals in any circumstances other than culturally acceptable bathing of a young child; or

Five

(c)   the child has been induced to touch the older person's breasts or genitals; or

(d)   there has been deliberate exposure to the child of the older person's breasts or genitals other than incidentally in the course of bathing or dressing;

(e)   the child has been deliberately induced to expose breasts or genitals other than incidentally in the course of bathing or dressing;

(f)   there has been any other form of physical contact or exposure between the adult and child that has led either to experience definite sexual arousal. It is irrelevant whether or not the child has willingly engaged in the sexual acts.

Excludes: sexual abuse outside the family/household (6.4).

1.8   Other

Any abnormal intrafamilial relationship that meets the general criteria on type and severity for this category, but which cannot be coded under 1.0 to 1.4.

2   Mental disorder, deviance or handicap[2] in the child's primary support group

The family disorders that are included in this category are those that are likely to impinge adversely on the child in ways that constitute a potential psychiatric risk. In some cases those ways may require codings on other categories (e.g. intrafamilial discord) but in other cases they may not (e.g. as with the stigma sometimes associated with mental illness or with epilepsy). Either way, the family disorder should be coded here if it meets the specified criteria (plus other codes, if relevant).

The general criteria for this category are:

(i)   that there is a socially disabling disorder or handicap or deviant behaviour pattern in a member of the child's immediate family or household; and

(ii)   that this is of a type and severity likely to interfere with the child's life in a manner that creates a potential psychiatric risk. Such interference may take the form of social stigma, or impaired parenting, or restrictions on

---

[2]   The terms handicap, disability and impairment are used loosely in this section and are not intended to accurately reflect the restricted definitions of these terms given in the WHO, International Classification of Impairments, Disabilities and Handicaps.

the child's social life, or abnormal family relationships, or involvement of the child in abnormal behaviours, or disrupted child care, or socially embarrassing situations.

2.0   Parental mental disorder/deviance

This category includes any type of currently disabling parental psychiatric disorder, irrespective of whether or not the parent is receiving psychiatric treatment. To be coded, the child need not be in contact with the parent and it is irrelevant whether the parent is currently a member of the child's household. However, the parental disorder must have impinged on the child to an important extent. For the purpose of this category, a parent is taken to mean any adult in the child's household who takes any aspect of a parental role with respect to the child (irrespective of whether they are biologically related or legally expected to take a parental role).

Diagnostic guidelines

There is no clear dividing line between normality and psychopathology; many adults have periods of anxiety or depression or heavy drinking or minor delinquent acts that fall short of a socially disabling mental disorder. Moreover, there is no unambiguous demarcation between psychiatric disorder and social deviance. For the purposes of coding it is not necessary to make such diagnostic distinctions (as the impact on the child may be similar in either case). Nevertheless, it is necessary that the disturbance or deviance be associated with substantial impairment in one or more of the adult's main areas of social role functioning.

Thus, criminality would be included if it was persistent or recurrent, or if it resulted in prison or some other form of residential placement, or if it involved any acts of violence against people. Alcoholism would be included if it involved any medical complications (such as epileptic fits, delirium tremens or periods of amnesia), if it interfered significantly with the person's social life or led to periods off work or repeatedly being late for work. Schizophrenia would be included if there was any overtly abnormal behaviour (psychotic or nonpsychotic) or if there were continuing socially oddities or observable drug side effects in conjunction with medication. Affective disorders would be included if they were of a severity sufficient to cause a regularly noticeable impairment in the person's social role performance (as shown e.g. by time off work, not coping with shopping or household chores, being unable to participate in usual leisure activities, or inadequate care of the children). Ordinarily

Five

any disorder resulting in psychiatric care or treatment should be assumed to meet these criteria. Conversely, any disorder that did not result in the person seeking any kind of professional help (such as from the family doctor or a social worker or community worker) should be assumed to fall short of the severity threshold unless there is clear evidence of definite substantial social impairment. Markedly deviant social behaviour associated with substantially impaired or distorted behaviour should be included even though the diagnosis may not be clear. Thus, morbid jealousy that led to following or systematically checking on the other person, or persistently violent behaviour, or extreme social isolation might all be relevant if social impairment was involved.

It should be assumed that any mental disorder that is accompanied by definite social disability, and which occurs in a parent who has regular contact with the child, meets the criterion that there is a likelihood that it has significantly interfered with the child's life in ways that constitute a psychiatric risk. Conversely, however, definite evidence that a disorder/handicap in an immediate family member has interfered substantially with the child's life (as, for example, by social restrictions or abnormal/inadequate parenting or altered life pattern stemming from definite overt social stigma) would constitute grounds for coding (such interference being indirect evidence of social disability), irrespective of whether the child is in contact.

Excludes: homosexuality (if not associated with other forms of disturbance).

mental handicap (if not associated with other forms of disturbance) see 2.1.

2.1   Parental handicap/disability

This category covers all types of parental handicap/disability that are not included in 2.0. The general criteria are comparable. That is, two conditions must be met:

(i)   there is some parental condition of a severity that leads to impairment in one or more of the adult's main areas of social role functioning, and

(ii)   that this is of a type and severity likely to interfere with the child's life in a manner that creates a potentially psychiatric risk.

Diagnostic guidelines

Five main types of handicaps/disability are those most likely to fulfil the criteria for coding here:

(i)   mental handicap;
(ii)   serious sensory deficits (e.g. deaf mute or blind parent);
(iii) severe epilepsy;
(iv)   chronic physical disorder/disability (such as cerebral palsy or severe asthma);
(v)   life-threatening illness (as with cancer).

However, in order to be counted it is not sufficient for one or other of these handicaps/ disabilities to be present. In addition, there must be positive evidence that it has impinged on the child in ways likely to create a potential psychiatric risk. This may be shown by:

(a)   definite overt social stigma (as evident, for example, by the child avoiding bringing friends home, or not telling other people about the parent's disability, or being teased about the parent's problem); or
(b)   inadequate care or supervision of the child by the affected parent; or
(c)   impaired parenting as evidenced, for example, by lack of sensitivity to child's cues, inept handling of child's distress or oppositional behaviour, or restricted play/conversation; or
(d)   family discord and tension; or
(e)   socially odd or embarrassing behaviour; or
(f)   restriction of the child's social life; or
(g)   imposition of age-inappropriate responsibilities on the child.
       Excludes: parental handicap/disability that does not interfere significantly with the child's life

2.2   *Disability in sibling*
The same two general criteria as in 2.1 apply except that, here, they apply to a sibling rather than a parent. The types of disability are those covered in 2.0 and 2.1.

Diagnostic guidelines
In addition to meeting the criteria for the presence of some mental or physical disability/handicap in a sibling, it is necessary that there be definite evidence that it impinges adversely on the child. The chief ways in which this may be shown are:

(a)   restriction on the child's social life either because the child is embarrassed to bring friends home or because care of the handicapped sibling imposes limitations on the child's social activities; or
(b)   interference with the child's property as by disruption/damage to

Five

belongings or not being able to leave things in the open when the sibling is present; or

(c) reduction of or distortion of parent–child interaction or of family social activities because of parental involvement with the disabled sibling; or

(d) substantial embarrassment to the child because of the disabled sibling's disruptive/deviant behaviour in public situations; or

(e) teasing of the child by peers regarding the sibling's oddities/handicaps; or

(f) physical intrusion of the child as by sharing the bed with an enuretic sibling or by being subjected to aggressive behaviour; or

(g) imposition of age-inappropriate responsibilities for care of the disabled sibling.

Excludes: disability of sibling that does not interfere significantly with the child's life.

2.8 *Other*

Any mental disorder, deviance or handicap that is present in a member of the child's household other than a parent or sibling, and which meets the two key criteria for the general category.

3 Inadequate or distorted intrafamilial communication

There are major difficulties in the assessment of intrafamilial patterns of communication and the research findings on associations between distorted communication patterns and psychiatric disorder are somewhat inconsistent. Many workers consider that communication features cannot be evaluated from the account of informants; rather it is necessary to observe families talking together. Even so there is a widespread belief, and some supporting evidence, that impaired family communication does constitute a psychiatric risk factor. The patterns of dominance, the amount of talk, the linguistic precision or clarity of communications, and the articulateness of family members do not seem particularly important. Rather, the crucial aspects of distorted intrafamilial communication concern confusing and contradictory messages, fruitless disputes, and a failure to use intrafamilial communication effectively to deal with family dilemmas, problems or conflicts. A further feature may be the maintenance of family secrets, or concealment of key information from the child that is needed for adaptive functioning.

Diagnostic guidelines

Distorted intrafamilial communication will tend to be characterized by:

(a) messages that are markedly contradictory in content and/or conflicting in the emotions expressed in the verbal content and those evident in the tone of voice or facial expression; or

(b) a marked tendency to talk at length at no-one in particular without responding to whatever has been said by other family members; or

(c) fruitless disputes that fail to end in resolution or agreement; or

(d) maladaptive concealment of key family information (as, for example, not telling a child that he is adopted); or

(e) regularly dealing with family difficulties by denial or refusal to face or discuss them.

Families vary greatly in their styles of communication and there are major cultural variations in the extent to which there is an expectation that families discuss issues that concern them. Distorted intrafamilial communication should be coded only if:

(i) it is clearly outside broadly defined normal limits for the child's subculture; and

(ii) the distorted or inadequate communication patterns are persistent and pervasive in so far as they involve the child; and

(iii) the poor communication is maladaptive in its effects (i.e. it leads family members to take inappropriate action, not to deal with crucial matters, or to fail to resolve important family issues).

4 Abnormal qualities of upbringing

This category covers certain qualities of upbringing by parents or other caregivers in the household such as a grandparent, foster parent, nanny, or older sibling that are abnormal in ways that are likely to constitute a psychiatric risk for the child.

Normal parenting involves many different dimensions, some of which are covered by other categories. Thus, for example, parenting involves a relationship between parent and child; abnormalities on this dimension are coded under '1'. Also it involves social-problem-solving, aspects of which are covered by category '3' (inadequate or distorted intrafamilial communication). In addition, however, parents are responsible for ensuring that children have appropriate and adequate learning experiences. It is abnormalities on that dimension that are primarily included in this category of abnormal qualities of upbringing. The first subcategory 'parental overprotection' deals with a style of parenting that serves to prevent children from having adequate opportunities for autonomy and responsibility and for relationships outside the parent–child dyad(s). The second subcategory covers situations in which the parents are failing to exercise the supervision necessary to prevent the child getting into psychologically risky situations. The third deals with a lack of the play and conversation that provide the immediate context and content of children's learning experiences from social interactions and from adult controlled or initiated activities. The fourth concerns parental pressures that serve to shape the child's activities in a direction that is socioculturally deviant and/or is discrepant with the child's own interests, abilities, and developmental level.

There are considerable sociocultural variations in patterns of child rearing and the categories here should be applied only when the quality of upbringing is definitely deviant in degree or type *and* when it is of a type likely to create a psychiatric risk for the child (such a risk includes liability to specific or general developmental delay). Ordinarily, a pattern that is acceptable within the child's own subculture (or religious group) would not be regarded as deviant even if it differed from the broader culture within which it was embedded. However, it should be coded if the pattern is one that definitely puts the child at psychiatric risk (great caution should be exercised in making this judgement; it would not be sufficient for the clinician to consider that it *might* be maladaptive because it was so unusual in the broader society).

The abnormality of parenting should be assessed in relation to what is appropriate for the child's particular circumstances given his/her developmental level, behaviour, physical state and sociocultural situation. Children's needs are inevitably influenced by their own characteristics; an impulsive child is likely to need more supervision, an anxious child more support, and a mature child less direct control. Similarly, the kind of linguistic interaction helpful to a deaf child will differ from that needed for a hearing one. Also, it should be appreciated that there are very wide sociocultural variations in views on what is appropriate for child to do. The coding of abnormal qualities of upbringing should be restricted to situations that are manifestly sufficiently deviant to create the likelihood of an increased psychiatric risk for the child.

It is common for patterns of upbringing to be deviant in several different respects. For example, there may be both inadequate parental supervision and also family discord. In that case *both* should be coded. Also, if both are a result of some parental mental disorder, that should be coded as well. This is necessary in order to cover the wide variety of patterns of abnormality that may be present and to avoid arbitrary decisions on which aspect should have precedence. The coding of abnormal patterns of upbringing should be applied if this is shown by either parent, regardless of the quality or rearing by the other parent, provided that the abnormal upbringing constitutes a substantial part of the child's experiences at home. However, if the abnormality applies to only one parent–child dyad, consider if there is associated discord between parents (1.1) or inadequate intrafamilial communication (3).

Rearing by siblings should be coded here only if a sister or brother has an obvious care-giving position comparable with that of a social parent.

4.0 Parental overprotection

The term 'overprotection' has been used to mean rather different things by different writers. However, as used here, it refers to a pattern of upbringing in which one parent (most often the mother) uses the relationship and/or the pattern of discipline in such a way as to severely constrain the child's ability to develop or maintain other relationships, and/or to take age appropriate decisions/responsibilities. The key components of overprotective behaviour are:

(i) prevention of independent behaviour; and
(ii) infantilization.

Thus the parent(s) inappropriately takes decisions for the child, cushions the child against challenges/stressors instead of helping him/her to cope him/herself, babys the child in a fashion that creates dependency and prevents him/her taking on appropriate responsibilities, restricts all (or almost all) components of the child's social experiences outside of the overprotective dyad, and (usually) isolates the child from other sources of social influence.

The notion of developmentally inappropriate parental control of the child's activities (in a direction that fosters dependency and infantilization) is central to the concept. In some cases this is accompanied by undue indulgence of the child within the infantile role (as by complying with the child's fads and fancies and by tolerance of childish disruptive behaviour) but this is not invariable and it is not part of the definition. Often the overprotection is emotionally enveloping, as well as socially restricting, but there is considerable variation in the extent to which this is or is not accompanied by overt warmth. Frequently the overprotective parent has an abnormally great emotional investment in the relationship with the child but the category is defined in terms of the impact on the child and not the parental psychopathology or motivation (which is, in any case, varied).

Diagnostic guidelines
The coding requires the presence of both prevention of independent behaviour and infantilization (in both cases to an extent that is abnormal in relation to socioculturally accepted age norms).

Prevention of independent behaviour may be shown by:

(a)   restriction of recreational activities largely to those that are either undertaken with the parent or that involve parental oversight or supervision; and/or

(b)   undue control of the child's friendships; and/or

(c)   discouragement of the child spending nights away with friends or relations; and/or

(d)   fostering of exclusive parent–child activities that are age inappropriate in degree or kind; and/or

(e)   selection of the child's clothes or activities to a point well beyond sociocultural age norms; and/or

(f)   not allowing the child to take independent decisions; and/or

(g)   taking over from the child so that the child rarely has to deal with his/her own social difficulties (i.e. fighting the child's 'battles' for him/her); and/or

(h)   the child is inappropriately prevented from going to places for leisure activities that are outside the parent's control and/or sight.

Infantilization may be shown by:

(a)   dressing/washing the child beyond the age when it is age appropriate in the culture; and/or

(b)   going to bed with the child to allay anxieties/provide comfort; and/or

(c)   taking the child to and from school or other places rather than letting the child use public transport or school buses when it would be age appropriate to do so; and/or

(d)   unusually frequent and inappropriate checking on the child's activities through observing him/her on the playground or elsewhere; and/or

(e)   unusually frequent, or unusually intrusive, inappropriate checking on the child by contact with teachers or others; and/or

(f)   inappropriately ready recourse to doctors or to bed rest for minor physical complaints; and/or

(g)   not allowing the child to encounter/deal with age appropriate challenges/stressors; and/or

(h)   insisting on staying with the child in hospital or accompanying for interviews when this is not age-appropriate according to sociocultural norms; and/or

(i)   the child is inappropriately prevented from engaging in normal sporting activities (such as swimming or football or cycling) because of the supposed risks involved.

In order for parental overprotection to be rated, both prevention of independent behaviour and infantilization must be present to a pervasive degree as shown by fulfilling at least several of the examples above under each heading.

It is common for overprotection to be accompanied by excessive anxiety or solicitude for the child. However this is not part of the definition. If an abnormally high degree of parental anxiety is present in addition to the other features, consider whether there is evidence of an anxiety state of a severity to warrant coding under 2.0.

Excludes: parental anxiety unaccompanied by infantilization and prevention of
         independent activities.
         overprotection that is restricted to certain specific activities.
         overprotection that has arisen as a temporary response to an acute illness or other crises.

4.1 *Inadequate parental supervision/control*

This category concerns a marked lack of effective control or supervision of the child's activities as judged in relation to the child's maturity and sociocultural background. As children grow up, it is necessary for parents to exercise a degree of supervision over their children's activities, modifying the degree of control in relation to the children's experiences, capabilities and maturity in order that they may learn to take responsibility but yet not run an unacceptable risk of getting into psychologically damaging situations. Excessive control is coded under 4.0 and inadequate control here. There are marked sociocultural variations in the extent of control that is regarded as desirable and inadequate control should be coded only when its degree is such as to be both socioculturally abnormal and of a kind likely to be psychologically risky.

Five

In practice, inadequate control is best assessed by evidence on:

(i)   lack of parental knowledge on what the child is doing or where (s)he is (as this negates the possibility of effective control); and

(ii)   clearly ineffective, or poorly operated, or poorly sustained control strategies (for the same reasons); and/or

(iii)   lack of concern or of attempted intervention when the child is known to be in psychologically risky situations.

Diagnostic guidelines

Lack of parental knowledge on child's whereabouts and activities may be shown by:

(a)   parents usually do not know where the child is when (s)he is out of the home; and/or

(b)   parents usually do not know the names (or addresses) of the friends whose home the child visits, or where (s)he stays overnight; and/or

(c)   parents usually do not know when the child comes in at night; and/or

(d)   the child is often left unsupervised outside the home when it is age-inappropriate for this to happen; and/or

(e)   the child is often left alone at home when it is age-inappropriate for this to happen.

Ineffective parental control may be shown by:

(a)   a lack of recognizable rules/guidelines on what the child is and is not allowed to do; and/or

(b)   parental approval or encouragement largely as a result of the parent's mood state rather than the child's behaviour; and/or

(c)   disciplinary interventions expressed in imprecise general terms (e.g. 'oh do be good') rather than in explicit terms of what is expected of the child; and/or

(d)   discipline that is so inconsistent within/between parents that there is a lack of a predictable response to the child's misbehaviour; and/or

(e)   attempts at discipline that are abortive without any consistent 'follow-through' to determine that the outcome is as intended.

Lack of concern or intervention when the child is in psychologically risky situations may be shown by:

(a)   lack of action when the child is known to be mixing in groups that carry substantial psychological risks (as when a young girl is engaged in potentially amorous relationships with older males, or when a child is part of a serious drug/delinquency group, or when a child is involved in an incestuous relationship with another family member); and/or

(b) lack of action when the child him/herself is known to have engaged in behaviour that is likely to result in his/her getting into serious trouble (as, for example, with the taking of 'hard' drugs, or delinquent activities or carrying offensive weapons); and/or

(c) lack of action when the child is known to be in seriously physically risky situations (as with young children climbing on roofs, or playing in dangerous areas, or playing with dangerous substances).

In order to rate as showing inadequate parental supervision/control there must be definite persistent and pervasive problems in this aspect of parenting as shown in several different aspects of the child's life. That means that at least several examples above must be fulfilled and ordinarily it may be expected that there will be abnormal behaviour in at least two out of the three specific aspects of control. However, if marked abnormalities in one area result in overt and severe lack of control that will suffice for rating.

This lack of control must extend across many of the child's activities but it may be manifest by one or both parents.

4.2 *Experiential privation*

Children both learn skills and develop social relationships in the context of conversation, play and activities with their parents and with other family members (as well as with people outside the home). This category is concerned with a marked lack in these interactions. Traditionally this has usually been termed a lack of 'stimulation' but that is a misleading expression of what is needed, in that children learn from an active engagement with other people and with their environment generally. This category refers to a lack of that active engagement, as a result of parental action (i.e. restriction or prohibition) or inaction (i.e. a failure to provide the relevant opportunities) with respect to linguistic, social, perceptual and motor activities. This should be judged in relation to the child's developmental level and sociocultural situation.

Experiential privation is usually manifest by:

(i)   a lack of parent–child conversation/play; and/or
(ii)   a lack of activities outside the home; and/or
(iii) confinement in circumstances that markedly limit active engagement with people and/or objects; and/or
(iv)   a lack of toys or other objects suitable for play by the child.

Diagnostic guidelines

A lack of parent–child conversation/play may be shown by:

(a)   a marked lack of opportunities for the child to talk with family members because they are rarely together; and/or

(b)   the parents do not discuss with the child what (s)he is interested in or what activities (s)he is engaged in or is planning; and/or

(c)   (if a younger child) the parents rarely read to the child or listen to him/her reading; and/or

(d)   little, if any, social chat over the meal table or during other times when the family are together; and/or

(e)   the parents rarely play games with the child or have a rough and tumble or engage in other forms of playful interaction; and/or

(f)   such interactions as there are, are largely at the parents' initiative, there being a definite tendency to ignore or otherwise not respond to the child's overtures.

A lack of activities outside the home may be shown by:

(a)   a lack of joint outings or activities such as walks, trips to museums or galleries or journeys to other places; and/or

(b)   a lack of shared activities between parent and child (as with sport, music, hobbies, or household activities); and/or

(c)   a lack of opportunity to participate in age-appropriate tasks such as shopping or travel.

Confinement that markedly limits active engagement with the environment may be shown by:

(a)   child not allowed outside the home for play; and/or

(b)   child confined to a room(s) that lack opportunities for play or conversation; and/or

(c)   (if a young child) left for long periods on his/her own during waking hours; and/or

(d)   child forced to go to bed at such an inappropriately early hour that there is a lack of time with parents or other family members.

A lack of toys/objects suitable for play may be shown by:

(a)   failure to provide the child with age-appropriate objects for play. There is huge sociocultural variation in the extent to which toys are available to children and economic considerations may markedly limit such provision. However, except in dire poverty, objects of some kind can be made suitable for child play by suitable improvization. A wide definition of age-appropriate objects should be adopted but it should be expected that some kind of range of such objects should be available to the child on an age and socioculturally appropriate basis; and/or

(b)   potential availability of age-appropriate objects for play but a lack of effective opportunity to use them because they are locked away or otherwise prevented from being used.

Unlike most other categories, experiential privation should be rated on the basis of the *overall* home environment and not in terms of the dyadic interaction with any one parent or other family member. Privation should *not* be rated if there is a lack of interaction with one parent but generally satisfactory level of experience overall (however, the lack with one parent may signal the presence of abnormalities rateable on other categories).

Because children can gain adequate experiences from many sources, the experiential privation must be both marked and pervasive to be rateable. Ordinarily, this will mean that the situation will fulfil several examples on at least two out of the four sets of criteria. However, the category should be rated on the overall level of experiences and occasionally a very severe lack under one heading may warrant inclusion: however, this should be regarded as likely to be unusual.

4.3   Inappropriate parental pressures

This category concerns parental pressures that are disjunctive with the child's developmentally and socioculturally appropriate needs and wishes. The implication is that the parents are pressing the child inappropriately to be different from what (s)he is. Such pressures may be sex-inappropriate (as by dressing a boy in girls' clothes or vice versa), age-inappropriate (as by forcing an older child to dress or behave like a young one or vice versa), or person-inappropriate (as by forcing the child to seek achievements in activities that are out of keeping with his/her talents and wishes). The pressures may come from one or both parents but to be rateable they must be persistent, definitely inappropriate, and of such a degree or pervasiveness that they significantly interfere with the child's life. Pressures that derive from a culturally unusual family style (as with religious groups) would not ordinarily be rated as inappropriate. However they may be included if parental norms/practices are pressed inappropriately in the face of the child's desire to adopt the norms of the wider culture in which the family is living.

Five

Diagnostic guidelines

Sex inappropriate pressures may be shown by:

(a) persistently pressing the child to dress, behave, or engage in activities that are of a kind or style or fashions regarded in the culture as confined to the opposite sex; and/or

(b) persistently pressing the child to behave only in extreme sex typical ways that are characteristic of the child's sex but are of such an extreme sex-exclusiveness as to be well outside the norms of the subculture in which the family live; and/or

(c) persistently pressing the child inappropriately to behave in a homosexual fashion when the child's sexual inclinations are established as heterosexual, or the reverse.

Age-inappropriate pressures may be shown by:

(a) persistently pressing an older child to dress or behave or engage in activities that in that subculture are manifestly too young or too old for the child's developmental level; and/or

(b) persistently pressing, against his/her wishes, a child to take on responsibilities that are clearly inappropriately above his/her age and capabilities; and/or

(c) persistent inappropriate discussing of highly personal adult matters (such as marital or extramarital sexual activities) with a young child.

Person-inappropriate pressures may be shown by:

(a) persistently pressing a child to engage in activities (such as sports or music or academic work) that are out of keeping with the child's consistently expressed wishes and/or capabilities; and/or

(b) persistently pressing a child to engage in all absorbing activities that occupy so much time and energies that they are socially restrictive and which reflect the parents' ambitions rather than the child's interests/ambitions (as, for example, by forcing involvement in highly competitive sporting or artistic activities). For inappropriate parental pressures to be codeable they must be definitely abnormal in the family's sociocultural context, definitely inappropriate in relation to the child's characteristics and they must be persistent and pervasive. However, they may be applied by only one parent and they may be present in only one of the three categories of inappropriateness (age, sex, and person).

Excludes: special encouragement of talents that are not exclusively restrictive;

complying with the child's wishes to engage in highly competitive activities that intrude into his/her social life;
encouraging the child to take on responsibilities that are ordinarily associated with an older age group but which the
child accepts and manages successfully.

4.8 Other

Other abnormal qualities of upbringing that do not fulfil the criteria for
4.0–4.3 situations should only be included when they interfere with
appropriate and adequate learning experiences for the child, and are
manifestly sufficiently deviant to constitute a psychiatric risk for the
child

5 Abnormal immediate environment

This category covers various aspects of the social or physical structure
of the child's environment that predispose to an adverse psychosocial
situation that creates a potential psychiatric risk. Necessarily the effects
on the child are likely to be less direct than with most of the other categories, but they are included here because of the evidence of risk. In the
absence of firm knowledge on the precise mechanisms that mediate the
risk, however, the coding should be based on the presence of the specified structural variable, and not on any judgement about actual damage
to the particular child.

The general criteria for this category are that:

(i)   the social/physical structure of the child's immediate environment is
      markedly atypical for the sociocultural setting;
(ii) the atypicality is of a type liable to create a disadvantageous or deviant
      psychosocial situation; and
(iii) there are empirical grounds for supposing that this situation provides a
      psychiatric risk for children.

5.0 Institutional upbringing

This category covers all situations in which the care of the child is provided on a residential basis in an institutional setting where there is
group, rather than family, care. In this connection, group care means that
children are looked after by a large number of adults on a shared care
basis (i.e. care-givers have scheduled free time when the care is taken
over by someone else). This contrasts with family care in which children

live with one or more adults who provide round-the-clock care without scheduled time off-duty (although alternative care-givers may be used on a frequent basis). Family care rarely involves regular night-time care by non-family members whereas group care usually does so.

Most forms of institutional upbringing involve a degree of roster caregiving; i.e. a pattern of rotating care-givers who have periods 'on' and 'off' duty. In some instances this may involve a very large number of adults in the care of any one child. This lack of continuous parenting by a relatively small number of adults who are regularly available to the child constitutes the most obvious difference from family care and this feature is thought by many to provide the main psychiatric risk.

The circumstances that give rise to an institutional upbringing include:

(i)   group foster care in which parenting responsibilities are largely taken over by some form of institution; such as residential nursery, orphanage, or Children's Home; or

(ii)   therapeutic care in which the child is in a hospital, convalescent home or the like without at least one parent living in with him/her.

Diagnostic guidelines
An institutional upbringing should be coded if:

(a)   parenting has been provided on a residential group, shared care basis in terms of group foster care, custodial care or therapeutic care (irrespective of whether the child is or is not accompanied by siblings); and

(b)   such care has lasted throughout the week (with or without weekends with parents); and

(c)   such care has been provided on a year-round basis (with or without holidays with parents) without regular prolonged vacation periods (as would be the case, for example, with boarding schools); and

(d)   it has lasted at least 3 months.

Excludes: family foster care (code 5.1)
              termly boarding school placement
              therapeutic care on a family basis in which the child lives with at least one parent
              institutional care lasting less than 3 months (but consider whether the criteria for 6.1 are met)
              all forms of non-residential day care
              custodial care in which the child is in some form of penal or welfare institution as a result of delinquent or quasidelin

quent activities; such as a reformatory, group home for delinquents, Borstal, detention centre or prison (code 9.0) therapeutic care for any form of psychiatric disorder (code 9.0)

5.1 Anomalous parenting situation

This category covers a somewhat heterogeneous range of situations that differ from the traditional norm of rearing by two biological parents. With many such situations there is empirical evidence of statistical associations with an increased psychiatric risk, although usually the increase in risk is relatively small. This applies, for example, to single parent families, adoptive parents, step-parents, foster parents, rearing of illegitimate children by others than their biological parents and a lack of a stable parental cohabiting relationship. In at least some of these cases it is likely that the risk stems from the psychosocial circumstances that give rise to the situation as much as to the situation itself (for example, this might be so with family foster care). Accordingly, for the most part, the situations constitute risk indicators rather than risk mechanisms.

In addition to the situations with an empirically demonstrated psychiatric risk (albeit often small), a few other situations are included in which evidence on the presence or absence of risk is meagre or unavailable. They are included (for the present) because of their marked atypicality and the presence of characteristics that seem to have parallels with those in the known risk situations. These situations of uncertain risk comprise rearing by a homosexual parent, group rearing in a commune where there is no immediate family context, rearing by a couple in which the mother has received artificial insemination by donor, and upbringing by relatives other than parents.

Diagnostic guidelines

Anomalous parenting situations include the following:

(i) foster family care by non-relatives;

(ii) upbringing by relatives other than parents (such as grandparents, aunts, older sibling, etc);

(iii) upbringing by a single parent in a non-cohabiting relationship (with or without the presence of other kin in the household); such single parenthood may be a result of the mother being unmarried, divorced, separated, or widowed;

(iv) upbringing of an illegitimate child by a couple who are not its biological parents (i.e. exclude children who are legally illegitimate but who are nevertheless reared by cohabiting biological parents),

Five

(v)   rearing by step-parents; i.e. any situation in which one parent is cohabiting with a partner who is not the biological parent of the child;

(vi)   rearing by adoptive parents (irrespective of whether the child knows that (s)he is adopted);

(vii) rearing by parents who are living in a non-familial context in a commune in which the parenting is shared with others, without the biological parents having a clearly demarcated exclusive parental role;

(viii) rearing by mother when the conception was by artificial insemination from a donor (irrespective of whether the child is aware of the fact);

(ix)   rearing by homosexual couple (male or female);

(x)   rearing by a couple in which one parent is overtly actively homosexual;

(xi)   rearing by a couple who lack a stable cohabiting relationship (i.e. there are repeated separations or changing partners without a consistent parent dyad)

(xii) any other situation in which rearing is other than by two cohabiting biological parents.

To be included the anomalous parenting situation must have lasted at least 3 months (however, for shorter duration one of the acute life events categories may apply and coded under '6').

Excludes: communal upbringing in which parents provide an exclusive family rearing that is complemented by day care by others (e.g. most kibbutzim)

rearing by cohabiting biological parents whose household is shared with other kin or non relatives

rearing by cohabiting biological parents of a legally illegitimate child

5.2   *Isolated family*

There is evidence that families function better when the parents experience social support from people outside the family with whom they have harmonious, confiding relationships. Also there is evidence that children gain from social experiences outside the family. It has been observed that some families having psychosocial problems with their children appear very socially isolated and, as an extension of these findings, it has been supposed that extreme social isolation may constitute a psychiatric risk factor for children. This category aims to provide coverage for situations characterized by such extreme social isolation.

The key defining feature is that the family as a whole has cut itself off from positive social contacts, or has been cut off by others as a result of their behaviour. There may or may not be adversive interactions with other people in the neighbourhood, or with social agencies. However, the situation is defined in terms of the *lack* of positive social interactions, and the presence or absence of negative interactions is irrelevant for the coding. To be codeable, however, it is necessary that the social isolation include the children (except in so far as they have social contacts at school).

The isolation may have arisen for a variety of different reasons. These include: paranoid ideation shared by both parents; a closed family system characterized by rigid personal attitudes that differ from those prevailing in the subculture; isolation brought about as a result of fear of discovery of some family secret; isolation stemming from the abnormal personality of the parents; and isolation by the neighbours because the family's behaviour is felt to be offensive or discreditable in some way.

Diagnostic guidelines
The essential criteria for the coding of family isolation are four-fold:

(i) lack of harmonious social contacts outside the home;
(ii) lack of visitors to the home;
(iii) lack of parental friendships; and
(iv) the extension of this social isolation to include the children.

A lack of harmonious social contacts outside the home will be shown by:

(a) a lack of participation in any group social activities (such as Church or social or sporting club), other than very infrequently; and
(b) a lack of shared outings with non-kin (or relations outside the immediate family) other than very infrequently; and
(c) a lack of regular informal positive social interactions with others with whom they have a persisting friendly relationship, other than very infrequently (however, there may or may not be casual conversations with people with whom they lack a persisting relationship in public settings, such as drinking places; typically such interactions by members of isolated families lack knowledge even of the names of the other people with whom they talk).

A lack of visitors to the home will be shown by:

(a) a failure to invite other people to the home, other than very infrequently; and
(b) a discouragement to uninvited visitors, other than very infrequently; and
(c) a lack of 'dropping-in' relationships with other people.

A lack of personal friendships will be shown by:

(a) a lack of confiding relationships with anyone outside the immediate family; and

(b) a lack of regular shared activities with anyone outside the immediate family.

The extension of this social isolation to include the child will be shown by:

(a) a prohibition on the child having visitors to the home, other than very infrequently; and

(b) a prohibition on the child visiting the homes of other people, other than very infrequently.

The essence of the category lies in the pervasiveness of the social isolation; hence it is necessary that all four criteria are met and that within each criterion there be no significant exceptions in terms of enduring relationships or positive social activities with people outside the family (other than those initiated by the child when outside the family confines, as at school). However, neither formal nor casual contacts that lack both shared activities and confiding should exclude the coding.

Excludes: restrictions on the child's social contacts that are not part of a general family social isolation (but consider coding 4.0); confinement of social contacts to those sharing a particular religious or cultural view; isolation resulting from membership of a discriminated group (code 7.0).

5.3 *Living conditions that create a potentially hazardous psychosocial situation*

There is evidence that markedly poor living conditions make good parenting more difficult and also create stresses for parents as individuals; however, there is a lack of consistent data on whether such living conditions create a psychiatric risk for children that is independent of the effects on parents. Moreover, there are immense difficulties in the establishment of criteria for 'poor living conditions' as these vary so enormously from country to country and even within any one country. Accordingly, this category is defined in terms of living conditions that create a potentially hazardous psychosocial situation, rather than directly in terms of level of poverty or lack of household facilities. In so far as housing disadvantage or low income have effects on parents or on parenting, they will be taken account of by other categories on this psychosocial axis. This category is confined to those living conditions that lead to a psychosocial situation that is not covered by other categories but which is likely to create a potential psychiatric risk.

Such living conditions fall into two main categories:

(i)   those that provide maladaptive constraints on interactions within the family;
(ii)   those that are associated with maladaptive effects outside the family.

In each case the criterion is that the circumstances lead to patterns that are both atypical for the culture and of a kind likely to constitute a psychiatric risk.

Diagnostic guidelines
Maladaptive constraints on family interactions may be shown by:

(a)   lack of sleeping space such that two or more opposite sex post-pubertal children have to share a nonpartitioned room; or
(b)   lack of sleeping space such that a child has to share the parental bed or bedroom beyond an age when it is considered appropriate to do so in the family subculture; or
(c)   'half way' housing, or other temporary accommodation, that necessitates a break-up of the family.

Maladaptive effects outside the family may be shown by:

(a)   'half way' housing or other temporary accommodation that necessitates the family sharing living space with other families; or
(b)   'half way' housing or other temporary accommodation that carries a public stigma in the subculture; or
(c)   lack of income, or inefficient use of income, such that children go to school in clothes that are regarded as odd or inadequate in the subculture to the extent that they constitute a source for personal shame or teasing by others; or
(d)   lack of income, or inefficient use of income, such that children are not able to participate in activities that would be regarded as generally expected in the subculture.

Excludes: housing limitations that force a child to share a room with a sick or disturbed relative (code under 2)

living conditions that cause malnutrition (code under appro
priate somatic disorder category)

poor living conditions that do not have psychosocial maladaptive effects of a kind likely to constitute a psychiatric
risk.

5.8   *Other*

Other living conditions that meet the general criteria for abnormal
immediate environment but which do not fulfil the criteria for 5.0 to 5.3.

6   Acute life events

Acute life events seem most likely to predispose to, or precipitate, psychiatric disorder if they are inherently unpleasant and if either they bring
about an adverse long-term change in life circumstances or, alternatively, they lead to a long-term impairment in individuals' views of themselves. In addition, it seems that unusual, extremely frightening or
humiliating experiences may also have long-term sequelae if the short-
term psychological traumata are sufficiently severe. This overall category comprises a grouping of somewhat different life events that have in
common the likelihood that they carry a substantial psychiatric risk.

It is *not* intended that the listing of life events should constitute a
comprehensive inventory of events that may have a significant psychological impact in individual cases. It is known that the impact is likely to
be influenced by a variety of personal circumstances. Thus, being elect-
ed sports team captain may be felt as rewarding by most children but
threatening to young people who doubt their ability to cope with the
added responsibilities. Such individual appraisals may be crucial in clinical formulations of psychosocial influences but inevitably they are outside the scope of a general classification that is to be used in routine
practice, rather than in systematic research that may provide sufficient
data for such judgements to be made reliably.

Unless there is some special feature that constitutes marked contextual threat, *normative* events are not included as stressors. By normative
events is meant those that are naturally expectable in the subculture.
These would include, for example: starting or leaving school, taking
school or national exams, birth of a sibling, and an older sibling leaving
home to get married, etc. The reasons for exclusion are that their
explanatory power is bound to be very low because such events occur to
almost everyone and that the empirical evidence suggests that their asso-

ciation with psychiatric disorder is very weak (if present). Accordingly, normative events are included only if there is something unusual about them that constitutes a high degree of contextual threat.

A further exclusion from this category is the group of events that have been brought about by the children themselves. Thus, a Court appearance may well be a stressful experience for delinquents but it cannot usefully be conceptualized as an independent potentially causal factor for psychiatric disturbance; similarly parental anger in response to a child's school refusal may be stressful but it is not separate from the child's own disorder or *independent* in the sense of not being a consequence of the child's own behaviour (but consider coding under 9).

Thus, the events that are to be coded comprise independent events that have occurred in the specified time period and that have been followed by a significant worsening of the child's life situation or have been associated with a serious long-term life psychological threat to the person's self concept, or have involved such a degree of danger or life disruption that a relatively lasting sense of fear or insecurity may be anticipated.

6.0 Loss of a 'love' relationship

It is a characteristic of human beings from the second half of the first year of life onwards that they form close affectionate ties with other people, that these ties provide important emotional support, and that the loss of such important ties constitutes a significant psychological stressor. In order for 'loss' to be coded it is necessary that it involve a relationship that is sufficiently emotionally close to carry the potential for confiding and psychological support. Ordinarily, this would apply to all parent–child relationships (even if they also included strongly negative components) and to important love relationships during adolescence. It might also apply to relationships with other adults (if they are caregivers in or outside the family or if they are seen by the child on a frequent or regular basis and are used for emotional comfort or support). The same might apply to siblings or especially close friends if there was clear evidence that they were used for comfort or support or if the relationships involved mutual confiding.

The second criterion needed for coding is that the child perceive significant loss. The loss may be total and permanent as by the death of the loved person; or it may be partial and semipermanent as by the greatly reduced contact with the parent who does not have child custody after divorce. In both these instances it may be assumed that the loss will be felt by children of all ages even though the way children respond may vary by developmental level. However, it is likely that the extent to which temporary separations are perceived as a loss will be a function of age to a large extent. Other children are usually able to understand that a period of absence will not be permanent and will be able to maintain a relationship while the loved person is away; that is much more difficult for young children.

Diagnostic guidelines

Loss should be coded only if it involves an emotionally close relationship and if the degree of loss is sufficiently great to carry a substantial psychiatric risk for most children of the same age living in the same circumstances. Loss should be regarded as significant if:

(a) there is death of a person fulfilling the role of social parent (irrespective of whether that person is still part of the child's household; however it is necessary that there has been sufficient contact in the recent past for it to be likely that the child continue to perceive the person as a social parent); or

(b) permanent or semi-permanent departure from the home of a social parent as a result of divorce, separation or other form of family break-up (irrespective of whether or not there is continuing non-custodial access); or

(c) temporary but lasting departure from the home of a social parent as a result of illness, working in another part of the country or any other factor, provided that it is likely from the child's age and/or circumstances that the separation will be perceived as a loss (ordinarily, for example, that may be assumed with absences of longer than a month with a preschool child); or

(d) death of a sibling (provided that the sibling shared the child's household or that there is evidence that the relationship is both close and supportive); or

(e) permanent or semi-permanent departure from the home of sibling in circumstances likely to be perceived as involving a major loss (for example, a sibling being removed to foster-care would count as a loss whereas a sibling leaving home to go to boarding school or to get married would not); or

(f) death of a special friend who has been seen on a frequent and regular basis by the child and for whom the relationship has involved emotional support or confiding; or

(g)   death or permanent loss of an adult outside the home whom the child sees regularly and frequently and with whom the child has a close loving relationship involving the child's confiding or receipt of emotional support; or

(h)   death of a loved pet with whom the child has a close relationship (this is likely to apply with a dog but probably would not with a pet bird; however the extent to which there has been a major relationship should be judged on the basis of the extent to which there has been playful interaction and emotional investment); or

(i)   a major rejection by anyone with whom the child has a manifestly close, loving relationship (for example a rebuff from a friend would not ordinarily count as a major rejection but the break-up of an intense love relationship in adolescence probably would count); or

(j)   miscarriage of a wanted pregnancy (code 6.3 for unwanted one); or

(k)   still-birth or death of an offspring of the child.

Excludes: loss resulting from the child's admission to a foster home or other institution (6.1) or loss resulting from an altered pattern of family relationships (6.2).

6.1   Removals from home carrying significant contextual threat

There is evidence that children's admissions to residential institutions frequently constitute significant psychosocial stress experiences. However, the extent to which admissions serve as stressors varies according to circumstances and according to the age of the children. In part, the stress stems from the loss or interruption of love relationships that is involved in the child's removal from home; in part from the lack of continuous emotionally involved care-giving that may be a consequence of institutional care; in part from the rebuff or rejection that may be implied in some forms of removal from home; and in part from unpleasant or adverse experiences in the new setting (as, for example, with some hospital admissions). Younger (especially preschool) children are more likely to experience major stress as a result of removal from home (as with hospital admission) both because they are less able to maintain love relationships over a period of absence and because they are less able to understand what is happening and why it is necessary. On the whole, very short admissions to hospital (less than a week) do not constitute a significant threat but admissions to a foster home or children's home of any duration tend to carry significant threat because of the greater implicit message of rejection. Single admissions to hospital may lead to immediate short-term distress but it is only repeated-admissions (when at least one previous admission has been during the pre-school years) that carry a significant psychiatric risk. Removal of a child to foster care may have been undertaken because of appropriate concerns about parental abuse or neglect; nevertheless if the child has had any sort of attachment relationship with the parents the removal is likely to have involved a significant element of threat (in spite of a reduction in overall adversity).

Diagnostic guidelines

Removals from home should be considered to carry significant contextual threat if there has been:

(a)   admission of any duration to a foster home or children's home (but exclude admissions as a consequence of the child's own deviant behaviour; code 9.1); or

(b)   admission to hospital for the second time, there having been one or more previous admissions during the preschool years (but exclude admission for psychiatric disorder; code 9.1).

> *Excludes*: a single admission to hospital (if this has involved a personal frightening experience, however, this may be coded as 6.5 see below),
> a period away from home that does not carry significant contextual threat (as, for example, with a prolonged holiday or a stay with relatives or convalescence after a physical illness)
> removals from home as consequence of the child's own deviant behaviour (code 9.1).

6.2   *Negatively altered pattern of family relationships*

For the most part risk factors stemming from abnormal patterns of family interaction or relationships are covered by category 1. However, this category (6.2) provides a means of coding *major adverse changes* in the child's pattern of relationships within the family that have been brought about by the entry into the family of some new person who, in some sense, seriously detracts from or constitutes a rival for the child's existing love relationships. Thus, the coding requires that two criteria be met:

(i)   there has been the arrival of a new person into the family; and

(ii)   this arrival has resulted in a major negative change in the child's pattern of relationships within the family.

The two commonest situations where these criteria apply are parental remarriage involving the entry into the family of a step-parent and the birth of a younger sibling. Neither should automatically be regarded as relevant; in order to be coded there must be evidence that the new person's entry has resulted in a significant adverse change in the child's relationships within the family (usually with one of the parents or principle care-givers).

Diagnostic guidelines

Parental remarriage would meet the criteria for an altered pattern of family relationships if it was accompanied by:

(a) a major reduction in parent–child interaction; or

(b) a relative lack of availability of the parent for emotional support; or

(c) a major change in the family pattern of communication/interaction, of discipline or of child rearing; or

(d) the assumption by the step-parent of a parental role before establishing a stable relationship with the child; or

(e) the entry into the home of step-siblings who detracted from the closeness of the original parent–child relationship.

The same might apply when a divorced/separated parent established a new love relationship that did not involve marriage; the relevance should be determined by the criteria as outlined for parental marriage. Equally, the entry into the home of a step-sibling would be relevant if this adversely affected the existing family relationships, even though the arrival did not coincide with a parental remarriage.

The birth of a sibling would meet the criteria if the birth was accompanied by any of criteria (a) to (e) for parental remarriage. Typically the birth would be relevant when there has been an increase in negative parent–child confrontations, an exclusion of the child from the care of/or interaction with the new baby, and/or a marked diminution in the availability of the parent for emotional support or play/conversation with the child.

The entry of other new members into the household may be relevant if they fulfil the above criteria. Thus, coding should be considered, for example, when a baby/child is adopted, when the parent accepts a foster-child, or when an older sibling re-enters the household with their own offspring. The essential criteria are not the degree of change as such but rather the extent of adverse alterations in the child's existing pattern of family relationships.

Five

6.3   Events resulting in loss of self-esteem

A sense of one's own value or worth is an important part of adaptive personality development and a major loss of self-esteem constitutes a significant psychosocial stressor that involves serious threat. Such a loss of self-esteem may be brought about by:

(i)   the child's failure in some specific task in an area involving high personal investment; or

(ii)   the disclosure or discovery of some personal or family event or feature that is perceived by the child as shameful or stigmatizing; or

(iii)   serious public humiliation; or

(iv)   the serious loss of trust in or respect for a loved person on whom the child relies for emotional support; or

(v)   the loss of self-respect that may be associated with an unwanted pregnancy (whether carried to term or terminated).

The key unifying features of the events that meet the criteria for this category are that they involve a change that is likely to bring about a major negative self reappraisal by the child.

Diagnostic guidelines

Task failure may be regarded as relevant if:

(i)   the failure is major either in terms of its effect on the child's progression in some activity/area of functioning or of its impact on the child's self-image; and

(ii)   the failure is in an area that involves the child's high personal investment; and

(iii)   the failure is likely to be perceived as implying the child's own lack of competence or capacity. Thus, failure in an internal school examination would be unlikely to meet these criteria; failure in a public examination would meet the criteria only if success was important to the child either because of his/her own investment in it or because success was necessary for some desired career progression. Failure in some non-scholastic area (such as music or sport) should be judged according to the same set of criteria. Dismissal from a job or forced redundancy would usually be considered to meet the criteria because of the loss of self-esteem involved.

Disclosure or discovery of some shameful or stigmatizing feature may be regarded as relevant if it is likely to result in the child feeling seriously demeaned or devalued in his/her own self-appraisal. Obviously, whether or not any disclosure will have that effect will depend on personal, as well as subcultural, norms and expectations. However, events that should be considered as possibly relevant would include discovery that:

(a) the child was illegitimate; or
(b) the parent was homosexual; or
(c) a parent, previously thought to be law-abiding, was a serious criminal; or
(d) the family could not cope (as by furniture being seized by the bailiffs or being thrown out of accommodation for non-payment of rent); or
(e) the child had become pregnant in circumstances that were likely to be felt as shameful in the subculture.

Public humiliation would be relevant if it involved, or was likely to involve, a major negative reappraisal of the child by friends, family, or other people of importance to the child. This might arise, for example, if the teachers at school publicly mocked the child's physical appearance or parent's extreme views or if the child was teased or bullied by peers in a way that led to public humiliation (if this involved violence that meets the criteria of 6.5, code both). Humiliation as a result of the child's own deviant behaviour should not be included here (code 9.2).

Events or happenings resulting in the child's loss of trust or respect for a loved person should be included if the loss was serious and if the person was someone on whom the child relied for emotional support. This might occur, for example, if the child discovered that the parents had told him/her, or acted on the basis of, a serious lie (such as pretending that the child was their biological offspring when in fact he/she had been adopted or fostered).

6.4 Sexual abuse (extrafamilial)

Epidemiological evidence suggests that sexual incidents involving children are an extremely common occurrence, so common that it is likely that most minor incidents are of little psychological significance. It is not known with any certainty which types of incidents are likely to be damaging. However, it may be presumed that the degree of psychiatric risk is influenced by the extent to which the incident directly involves or is focused on the child; by the degree and directness of personal (sexual) intrusion; by the abuse of power stemming from age, authority or personal/professional relationship; and by the extent of physical coercion or trauma.

Diagnostic guidelines

Sexual incidents should be regarded as constituting abuse if:

(i) the other person is substantially older than the child (i.e. it is not an equal love relationship in which the other person is technically an adult but in real terms is regarded by the child as an equal partner); and either

(ii) the sexual incident took place on the basis of the other person's position or status (e.g. she/he was the child's doctor or priest or professional care-giver outside the household), or

(iii) the child was an unwilling participant (irrespective of whether or not there was active resistance).

In addition, the coding of abuse requires that:

(a) there was contact or attempted contact with the child's breasts or genitals; or

(b) contact or attempted contact with the other person's breasts or genitals; or

(c) sexual exposure by the other person in which there was either attempted touching or close confrontations of the child (ie genital exposure at a distance or not specifically directed at the child would ordinarily be excluded); or

(d) the other person sought to undress the child (or get the child to undress) in circumstances in which this was socially unacceptable; or

(e) the other person enticed or sought to entice the child to go away with them (into a vehicle or to another place) in circumstances in which this carried psychological threat.

Excludes: sexual abuse within the family (1.4).

6.5   Personal frightening experiences

On the whole, the limited available evidence suggests that brief frightening experiences, however upsetting at the time, do not usually carry a significant long-term psychiatric risk. However, it seems likely that such experiences may carry a significant risk if the nature or context of the event is such as to carry an implicit or explicit threat with respect to the child's future well-being. Such threats may stem from the major uncertainties over possible serious consequences, from the actual damage to others, or from persisting trauma to the child.

Diagnostic guidelines

To be included, the experience must be clearly outside the realm of ordinary expectable happenings and must carry threat for the child's future.

Such threat may be manifest:

(a) in the serious uncertainties as to whether the child will survive unscathed (as for example may be the case with being kidnapped or held hostage even though, in the event, no harm resulted); or

(b) if there is a serious implicit threat to life (as for example with floods, earthquakes, volcanoes and other natural disasters resulting in death or serious injury to other people physically or emotionally close to the child even though the child is uninjured); or

(c) if the child is injured in ways that carry serious threats to the child's self image or security (as for example with the potential scarring implicit in a dog bite on the face, or with personal involvement in an accident that involves major damage to people or property); or

(d) if severe lasting pain is involved (as with an extensive severe burn); or

(e) if the child is a witness to severe accidental or deliberate trauma to members of the immediate family or other individuals with whom there is an emotionally close relationship (as with rape or violent assault or a serious road traffic accident); or

(f) if the child is personally involved in an episode involving threat to property in circumstances that carry personal threat as well (as, for example, with a burglary involving serious upheaval to the child's own room, or the child discovering a break-in to the home, or the child being mugged or being with an immediate family member who is mugged); or

(g) if the episode carries the likelihood of repetition/reoccurrence (e.g. with serious bullying at school or in the neighbourhood).

Excludes: natural disasters in which the child is not directly involved as above but which result in the death of someone close to the child (code 6.0);

disasters carrying potential threat to the family but not directly perceived by the child, as e.g. with a factory accident in the neighbourhood causing nuclear contamination (code only if there are elements that meet criteria for other categories)

civil unrest that does not directly impinge on the child in ways that carry long-term threat;

life events that impinge on family members but which do not directly involve the child (code only if the family reaction results in psychosocial situations that meet the criteria for other categories).

Five

6.8   *Other acute life events*
Any other acute life event, not covered by categories 6.0 to 6.5, which meets the general criteria for events carrying substantial long-term contextual threat (psychological or physical).

7   Societal stressors

This category covers stressors that reflect factors deriving from broader social or cultural forces or features, rather than characteristics of the child's own immediate environment or individualized experiences. To be included, the events, circumstances or happenings must impinge directly on the child and must carry a substantial degree of long-term psychological or physical threat.

7.0   *Persecution or adverse discrimination*
This category includes events or experiences that:

(i)   directly impinge on the child; and
(ii)   cause long-term threat; and
(iii)   involve persecution or adverse discrimination based upon the child's membership of some broader ethnic, religious or other group (rather than the child's own personal characteristics).

The coding should be restricted to events/experiences that result in:

(i)   physical damage; or
(ii)   exclusion from activities of importance to the child; or
(iii)   public stigma or humiliation that goes beyond the unpleasant behaviours that constitute part of a broadly defined range of ordinary expected life stresses.

Diagnostic guidelines
Persecution/adverse discrimination may include:

(a)   beatings up or physical degradations (such as soiling the child's clothes);
(b)   refusal to allow the child to participate in desired work or leisure activities;
(c)   forcing the child to be publicly labelled by means of clothing, having to sit or play in defined areas etc; or
(d)   any form of serious public stigma or humiliation.

In all cases it is necessary that discrimination be on the basis of the child's membership of some group (as defined by skin colour, religion, ethnic origin, etc.) rather than the child's own characteristics, appearance or behaviour. Teasing and name-calling that does not go beyond what might be expected as part of ordinarily unpleasant peer-group interactions would not be sufficient for coding; however, public humiliations as by a teacher's gross overt discriminatory behaviour should be included.

Excludes: bullying or teasing on the basis of personal characteristics (consider whether this meets the criteria for 6.5 or 6.3).

7.1   Migration or social transplantation
Such limited evidence as is available suggests that there is little psychiatric risk associated with geographical moves as such (involving home and/or school). However, there may be a significant risk if:

(i)   the move is degradingly forced (as with refugees or with eviction); or
(ii)   there is a major disruption of personal ties or relationships; or
(iii)   the move involves a change to a very different subculture; or
(iv)   the child is placed in an environment that requires the learning of a new language; or
(v)   the move results in a major loss of social status.

Diagnostic guidelines
Moves should be included if:

(a)   the child is removed to another environment without his/her family (as with certain forms of evacuation); or
(b)   the move of the family is forced and involves loss of personal security (as with being made a refugee or being evicted from the family home; do not include, however, moves that arise as a consequence of rehousing unless long-term threat is involved); or
(c)   the move involves a change to a radically different culture or one in which the child has to learn a new language (do not include if the child remains part of his/her own subculture as might be the case with diplomatic or military families); or
(d)   the move involves a major reduction in the child's well-being or social circumstances or social standing (as might be the case, for example, with a move following family bankruptcy).

Five

7.8   *Other*

Any other societal stressor, not covered by categories 7.0 and 7.1 that meets the general criteria for societal stressors.

8   Chronic interpersonal stress associated with school/work

Both school and work constitute social environments to which people are exposed for many of their waking hours. This category concerns abnormal relationships experienced within school or work that are of a kind and of a severity likely to constitute a psychiatric risk factor for young people. In that respect they constitute a parallel to the abnormal intrafamilial relationships covered by categories 1.0 to 1.8. The chronic interpersonal stress associated with school/work may stem from rejection by the peer group; from scapegoating of the person by school teachers (or supervisors at work); or from general unrest or discord at school/work.

The interpersonal stress must be *associated* with school or work in order to be applicable, but it need not necessarily be experienced on school or work premises, nor need it necessarily involve people at the child's own school or work. Thus, for example, regular bullying on the way to school by pupils from another school would be included.

As with abnormal relationships within the family, it will often be the case that the child's own actions, attitudes, or responses will have played a part in creating or prolonging the interpersonal difficulties at school or work. However, codings should be made solely on the basis of the abnormality in other people's behaviour, irrespective of the child's own contribution to the poor relationship.

8.0   *Discordant relationship(s) with peers*

This category concerns discord between the child and his/her peers. A lack of positive relationships is not sufficient for coding; there must be serious active negative interchange. Similarly, brief repeated episodes of quarrelling would not be sufficient; rather, the relationship(s) must be persistently and generally negative. A single markedly negative relationship of a kind that fulfils the diagnostic guidelines or multiple relationships of the same kind should both be included. As a general principle, the presence of discordant relationships should be coded regardless of compensating good relationships with others.

Diagnostic guidelines

Relationships with peers should be regarded as abnormal when the child is:

(a) repeatedly tormented or denigrated or insulted; or
(b) repeatedly threatened or bullied; or
(c) subjected to coercion to take part in activities against his/her will; or
(d) subjected to extortion; or
(e) actively rejected, ignored or isolated by his/her peers; or
(f) repeatedly subjected to humiliating experiences.

8.1 Scapegoating of child by teachers or work supervisors

This category refers to personally focused (or targeted) marked negative feelings of one or more teachers or work supervisors towards the child. The negative feelings must be specifically directed towards the child but it is possible for the scapegoating or hostility to apply to more than one child in the peer group.

Diagnostic guidelines

The coding requires that:

(i)   the negative adult behaviour is clearly abnormal in form and/or degree; and
(ii) it is specifically focused on the child as an individual; and
(iii) it is persistent over time and pervasive over several child behaviours (i.e. an excessive adult reaction to just one or two specific child actions would not be adequate for coding).

The hostility/scapegoating may be shown by:

(a) an unreasonable tendency to blame the child for problems or difficulties or wrongdoing in the school or work situation; or
(b) repeated criticisms of the child that extend to a general denigration of the child as a person, that generalize to past misdeeds, or which include a clear expectation of future misdeeds; or
(c) a general tendency to attribute the child with negative characteristics; or
(d) a clear tendency specifically to 'pick on' the child or to involve the child in negative interchanges when the adult is feeling miserable, irritable or bad-tempered; or
(e) treating the child unfairly in relation to other people in the school/work situation – with excessive work load or responsibilities, an exclusion from positive activities, or marked lack of attention to the child's needs or difficulties.

Five

8.2   Unrest in the school/work situation

This category concerns discord or unrest in the school/work situation that impinges on the child to a marked extent but which is mainly characterized by discord between others rather than with the child him/herself. In order to be coded, the situation must be abnormal in the sociocultural context, it must have lasted for at least half of the time period used for rating, and it must have involved the child to a substantial extent. The unrest/discord may be mainly between other children, between adults at school/work, or between teachers and other pupils (or supervisors and other workers). To be coded it should be of a degree to interfere with the child's task involvement or interpersonal relationships in the school/work situation.

Diagnostic guidelines
The school/work situation should be regarded as abnormal if it is characterized by:

(a)   repeated or persistent disruptive behaviour with frequent disputes, altercations, aggressive or destructive acts by adults or children or both; or

(b)   a marked lack of disciplinary control such that work activities cannot continue or that repeated assistance from others is required in order to regain control; or

(c)   frequent disputes or quarrels between teachers (work supervisors).

8.8   Other
Any other chronic interpersonal stress associated with school/work that meets the general criteria on type and severity for this category, but which cannot be coded under 8.0 to 8.2.

Excludes: stress resulting from scholastic failure or inadequate teaching or other non-social aspects of the school/work environment.

9   Stressful events/situations resulting from the child's own disorder/disability

This category is strictly limited to events/situations that result from the child's own disorder/disability (and hence cannot be coded under categories 1 to 8), but which nevertheless by their occurrence create a substantial additional stressor for the child. Thus, a child's placement in a residential institution may have been made on the basis of the child's disorder but yet the institutional upbringing might itself constitute an additional psychiatric risk factor. Similarly, a child might be excluded from school as a result of his/her own disruptive behaviour but still the exclusion could constitute a further significant stress factor. This category should be coded only if it is clear that the event/situation that resulted from the child's own disorder/disability did indeed constitute a substantial additional stressor.

As already noted, it is likely that the child's behaviour may have contributed in part to a variety of abnormal psychosocial situations. Thus, for example, this is probably so in many cases for discord in the family or at school. However, this assumption is not a reason for coding the situation here (see instructions for coding categories 1 to 8). Category 9 is restricted to events/situations where the child's role in bringing them about is both overt and major.

9.0 *Institutional upbringing*
Coding of this category should be made in accordance with the guidelines for 5.0, with the additional requirement that the upbringing was mainly brought about by the child's own disorder/disability. Thus, upbringing in a psychiatric hospital or an institution for delinquents would be included here.

9.1 *Removal from home carrying significant contextual threat*
The criteria for rating this category are those already outlined for category 6.1, but with the additional requirement, the removal occurred primarily as a consequence of the child's own disorder/disability.

9.2 *Events resulting in loss of self-esteem*
Coding of this category follows the guidelines for category 6.3, but with the additional requirement that the event was primarily brought about by the child's own behaviour. Thus, the loss of self-esteem may stem from the public exposure of a shameful aspect of the child's behaviour; from the humiliation associated with expulsion from school or dismissal from work; or from the loss of trust or respect from someone important to the child as a result of something the child has done.

Excludes: loss of self-esteem resulting from discovery of shameful or stigmatizing facts about other family members (code 6.3).

9.8 *Other*
Any other event/situation carrying long-term contextual threat that meets the general criteria for category 9. This category should be used

Five

only when it is clear that the event/situation resulted from the child's own disorder/disability and that such event/situation created a substantial additional stressor for the child.

Acknowledgements

Field trials on the psychosocial axis were carried out in a number of centres, particularly a large group of such centres in Germany.

Athens (Greece)	Dr J. Tsiantis
Enschede (Netherlands)	Dr G.L.G. Couturier
Hong Kong (HK)	Dr T.P. Ho, Dr W.M. Kwok, Dr P. Lee, Dr F. Lieh Mak
Ljubljana (Slovenia)	Dr A. Kos
Nijmegen (Netherlands)	Dr P. van der Doef
Paris (France)	Dr E. Fombonne, Dr J. Laget, Dr G. Vila, Dr O. Halfon, Dr M.-L. Paillere-Martinot, Dr C. Aussilloux, Dr M.-C. Mouren-Simeoni, Dr B. Massari
Zurich (Switzerland)	Dr H.-Ch. Steinhausen

In Germany

Berlin	Professor U. Lehmkuhl
Berlin Herzberge	Dr A. Israel
Berlin Marzahn	Dr H. Schernikau
Erlangen	Professor R. Castell
Frankfurt/M	Dr R.D. Lehman
Heidelberg	Professor M. Müller-Küppers
Köln	Professor G. Lehmkuhl
Mannheim	Professor M.H. Schmidt (Univeristy of Heidelberg)
München	Professor J. Martinius
Riedstadt	Dr E. Meyer
Rostock	Professor R. Cammann

Axis Six

Global Assessment of Psychosocial Disability

This axis should reflect the patient's psychological, social, and occupational functioning at the time of the clinical evaluation. Except for very acute disorders, this should be assessed for the period of three months prior to the assessment, but the intention is that the coding reflects functioning during the period of disorder. The codings should concern the decrease in psychosocial functioning that has arisen as a consequence of psychiatric disorder (i.e. any disorder on Axis One), or a specific disorder of psychological development (i.e. any disorder on Axis Two), or mental retardation (i.e. a code of 70–79 on Axis Three). That due to physical (or environmental) limitations should not be coded. Rate the subject's lowest level of functioning during the last 3 months. Code on the basis of overt social functioning within the child's actual social context of opportunities without regard for the presence/absence of psychiatric symptoms.

The assessment of psychosocial disability should be based on the degree to which the child maintains relatively harmonious relationships with parents, siblings and teachers and other adults; keeps him/herself clean and tidy to a degree consonant with his/her age and social circumstances; performs reasonable household work tasks; is able to leave the home without difficulty; copes with school/class work in a manner consistent with his/her age and intelligence; forms reciprocal peer relationships that involve shared activities; engages in a range of spare time activities; and copes with paid jobs (if employed). The decision on whether the disability is due to psychiatric disorder should be based primarily on whether the change in level of psychosocial functioning shows a meaningful temporal relationship to the onset of psychiatric symptoms and on whether there is a plausible way in which the symptoms could have led to a psychosocial disability. It should be noted that this casual relationship of the disability only to mental factors coded in the first three axes, differs from the principle used in the WHO multiaxial classification for use in adult psychiatry, which allows for the coding of disability caused by both mental and physical disorders.

0   Superior/good social functioning
Superior/good functioning in all social domains. Good interpersonal relationships with family, peers and adults outside the family; effective

coping with all social situations encountered; and good range of leisure activities and interests.

1 *Moderate social functioning*
Moderate functioning overall, but with transient or minor difficulties in one or two domains only (functioning may, or may not be superior in one or two other domains).

2 *Slight social disability*
Adequate functioning in most domains but slight difficulties in at least one or two domains (such as manifested by difficulties in friendships, constrained social activities/interests, difficulties in family relationships, less than effective social coping, or difficulties in relationships with adults outside the family).

3 *Moderate social disability*
Moderate disability in at least one or two domains.

4 *Serious social disability*
Serious disability in at least one or two domains (such as marked lack of friends, or inability to cope with new social situations, or inability to attend school).

5 *Serious and pervasive social disability*
Serious disability in most domains.

6 *Unable to function in most areas*
Needs some ongoing supervision or care from other people in order to maintain everyday functioning; unable to manage completely on own.

7 *Gross and pervasive social disability*
Sometimes unable to maintain minimal personal hygiene, or sometimes requires continued close supervision to avoid danger to self or others, or gross impairment in all means of communication.

8 *Profound and pervasive social disability*
Persistent inability to maintain personal hygiene or persistent risk of severe hurting self or others or total lack of communication.

Acknowledgements

Many individuals and organizations contributed to the production of the classification of the mental and behavioural disorders in ICD-10, including those relevant to child and adolescent psychiatry. Field trials took place in some 40 countries, and the effort has been acknowledged in the full WHO publications presenting this classification. In view of the fact, however, that this publication is the first presenting the full text of Axis Five with its glossary and guidelines, it is appropriate to acknowledge here the large amount of work put into this by the WHO working group comprising Dr Gera van Goor-Lambo, Professor Fritz Poustka and Professor Sir Michael Rutter. Those centres that carried out field trials of the psychosocial axis are listed at the end of that axis. Dr John Orley, WHO Programme on Mental Health, had overall responsibility for co-ordinating the work on this multiaxial classification.

Index

Note: For those entries marked # see List of categories for additional fourth or fifth character. The letters NEC stand for 'not elsewhere classified'.

'specified NEC' indicates that a more detailed subclassification of this disorder is provided. The specific disorders are included elsewhere in the index but not always under the more general descriptor. In such cases reference should be made to the other entries at the same level of the index. If the condition is still not found then the relevant three-character category of the classification itself should be consulted in order to obtain more precise coding.

The roman numeral I, II, III, IV, or V which immediately follows each entry, indicates the axis to which that category belongs. In the case of axes I–IV, the category consists of a letter followed by numbers. For axis V, the categories consist only of numbers. No index entry is provided for Axis VI.